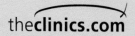

CLINICS IN PLASTIC SURGERY

Body Contouring After Massive Weight Loss

Guest Editor
AL ALY, MD, FACS

January 2008 • Volume 35 • Number 1

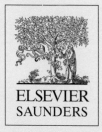

ELSEVIER
SAUNDERS

An imprint of Elsevier, Inc
PHILADELPHIA LONDON TORONTO MONTREAL SYDNEY TOKYO

W.B. SAUNDERS COMPANY
A Division of Elsevier Inc.

1600 John F. Kennedy Blvd., Suite 1800, Philadelphia, PA 19103-2899

http://www.theclinics.com

CLINICS IN PLASTIC SURGERY Volume 35, Number 1
January 2008 ISSN 0094-1298, ISBN-13: 978-1-4160-5053-7, ISBN-10: 1-4160-5053-1

Editor: Sarah Barth

Reprints. For copies of 100 or more, of articles in this publication, please contact the Commercial Reprints Department, Elsevier Inc., 360 Park Avenue South, New York, New York 10010-1710. Tel.: (212) 633-3813 Fax: (212) 462-1935, e-mail: reprints@elsevier.com.

The ideas and opinions expressed in *Clinics in Plastic Surgery* do not necessarily reflect those of the Publisher. The Publisher does not assume any responsibility for any injury and/or damage to persons or property arising out of or related to any use of the material contained in this periodical. The reader is advised to check the appropriate medical literature and the product information currently provided by the manufacturer of each drug to be administered to verify the dosage, the method and duration of administration, or contraindications. It is the responsibility of the treating physician or other health care professional, relying on independent experience and knowledge of the patient, to determine drug dosages and the best treatment for the patient. Mention of any product in this issue should not be construed as endorsement by the contributors, editors, or the Publisher of the product or manufacturers' claims.

Clinics in Plastic Surgery (ISSN 0094-1298) is published quarterly by Elsevier Inc., 360 Park Avenue South, New York, NY 10010-1710. Months of issue are January, April, July, and October. Business and Editorial Offices: 1600 John F. Kennedy Blvd., Suite 1800, Philadelphia, PA 19103-2899. Customer Service Office: 6277 Sea Harbor Drive, Orlando, FL 32887-4800. Periodicals postage paid at New York, NY and additional mailing offices. Subscription prices are $326.00 per year for US individuals, $472.00 per year for US institutions, $164.00 per year for US students and residents, $370.00 per year for Canadian individuals, $539.00 per year for Canadian institutions, $395.00 per year for international individuals, $539.00 per year for international institutions, and $195.00 per year for Canadian and foreign students/residents. To receive student/resident rate, orders must be accompanied by name of affiliated institution, date of term, and the *signature* of program/residency coordinator on institution letterhead. Orders will be billed at individual rate until proof of status is received. Foreign air speed delivery is included in all *Clinics* subscription prices. All prices are subject to change without notice. **POSTMASTER:** Send address changes to *Clinics in Plastic Surgery*, Elsevier Periodicals Customer Service, 6277 Sea Harbor Drive, Orlando, FL 32887-4800. **Customer Service: 1-800-654-2452 (US). From outside of the US, call 1-407-345-4000.**

Clinics in Plastic Surgery is covered in *Current Contents, EMBASE/Excerpta Medica, Science Citation Index, Index Medicus, ASCA, and ISI/BIOMED.*

Printed in the United States of America.

BODY CONTOURING AFTER MASSIVE WEIGHT LOSS

GUEST EDITOR

AL ALY, MD, FACS
Iowa City Plastic Surgery, Coralville, Iowa

CONTRIBUTORS

AL ALY, MD, FACS
Iowa City Plastic Surgery, Coralville, Iowa

ADEL BARK, MD
Iowa City Plastic Surgery, Coralville, Iowa

JOSEPH F. CAPELLA, MD
Department of Plastic Surgery, Hackensack
University Medical Center, Hackensack; and
Assistant Clinical Professor of Surgery, University
of Medicine and Dentistry of New Jersey, Newark,
New Jersey

ROBERT F. CENTENO, MD, MBA
Body Aesthetic Plastic Surgery & Skincare Center,
St. Louis, Missouri

MARK W. CLEMENS, MD
Resident, Department of Plastic Surgery,
Georgetown University Medical Center,
Washington, District of Columbia

ALBERT CRAM, MD, FACS
Iowa City Plastic Surgery, Coralville, Iowa

STEVEN P. DAVISON, MD, DDS, FACS
Associate Professor of Surgery, Department
of Plastic Surgery, Georgetown University
Medical Center, Washington, District of
Columbia

SUSAN E. DOWNEY, MD, FACS
Clinical Associate Professor of Surgery (Plastic),
Keck School of Medicine, University of Southern
California, Los Angeles, California

ANTHONY N. FABRICATORE, PhD
Department of Psychiatry, Center for Weight and
Eating Disorders, University of Pennsylvania
School of Medicine, Philadelphia, Pennsylvania

JOHN E. GROSS, MD
Assistant Clinical Professor of Surgery (Plastic),
Keck School of Medicine, University of Southern
California, Los Angeles, California

DENNIS J. HURWITZ, MD, FACS
Clinical Professor of Surgery (Plastic), University
of Pittsburgh Medical School; and Attending
Physician, Magee-Women's Hospital, Pittsburgh,
Pennsylvania

JEFFREY M. KENKEL, MD
Professor and Vice-Chairman, Department of
Plastic Surgery, The University of Texas
Southwestern Medical Center, Dallas, Texas

GERALD KHACHI, MD
Body Contour Fellow, Plastic and Reconstructive
Surgery, University of Pittsburgh, Pittsburgh,
Pennsylvania

ALEXANDER MANSUR, MD
Iowa City Plastic Surgery, Coralville, Iowa

DAVID W. MATHES, MD
Assistant Professor of Surgery, Division of Plastic
Surgery, Department of Surgery, University of
Washington School of Medicine, Seattle,
Washington

CONSTANTINO G. MENDIETA, MD, FACS
Coconut Grove, Florida

TIM NEAVIN, MD
Resident in Plastic Surgery, University of
Pittsburgh Medical Center, Pittsburgh,
Pennsylvania

DANIELE PACE, MD
Iowa City Plastic Surgery, Coralville, Iowa

J. PETER RUBIN, MD
Director, Life After Weight Loss Program, Plastic and Reconstructive Surgery, University of Pittsburgh, Pittsburgh, Pennsylvania

MATTHIAS A. REICHENBERGER, MD
Department of Plastic and Reconstructive Surgery, Dreifaltigkeits-Hospital, Wesseling, Germany

DIRK F. RICHTER, MD
Department of Plastic and Reconstructive Surgery, Dreifaltigkeits-Hospital, Wesseling, Germany

SILVIA CRISTINA ROTEMBERG, MD
Department of Plastic Surgery, Cleveland Clinic, Cleveland, Ohio

DAVID B. SARWER, PhD
Department of Psychiatry, Center for Weight and Eating Disorders; and Division of Plastic Surgery, Department of Surgery, The Edwin and Fannie Gray Hall Center for Human Appearance, University of Pennsylvania School of Medicine, Philadelphia, Pennsylvania

JEFFREY L. SEBASTIAN, MD
Assistant Clinical Professor of Surgery, David Geffen School of Medicine at UCLA, Los Angeles; and Private Practice, Santa Monica, California

SHEHAB SOLIMAN, MD
Lecturer of Plastic Surgery, Department of Surgery, Cairo University, Kasr El-Aini Hospitals, Cairo, Egypt

ALEXANDER STOFF, MD
Department of Plastic and Reconstructive Surgery, Dreifaltigkeits-Hospital, Wesseling, Germany

FERNANDO J. VELASCO-LAGUARDIA, MD
Department of Plastic and Reconstructive Surgery, Dreifaltigkeits-Hospital, Wesseling, Germany

RAMÓN VILA-ROVIRA, MD
Plastic Aesthetic Surgeon and Director, Institut Vila-Rovira, Centro Médico Teknon, C/Vilana, Barcelona, Spain

V. LEROY YOUNG, MD, FACS
Body Aesthetic Plastic Surgery & Skincare Center, St. Louis, Missouri

BODY CONTOURING AFTER MASSIVE WEIGHT LOSS

Volume 35 · Number 1 · January 2008

Contents

David B. Sarwer and Anthony N. Fabricatore

As bariatric surgery for extreme obesity continues to grow in popularity, so does interest in postbariatric surgery body-contouring surgery. There is an extensive literature on the psychological characteristics of persons with extreme obesity who undergo bariatric surgery and the psychological changes that typically occur postoperatively. Far less, however, is known about the psychological aspects of body contouring following massive weight loss. This article reviews the psychosocial characteristics of individuals with extreme obesity who undergo bariatric surgery, as well as the changes in these traits that typically occur postoperatively. Because there have been few studies of the psychological aspects of patients who have lost massive amounts of weight, we use related literatures on the relationship between body image dissatisfaction and other plastic surgical procedures to identify the most relevant research and clinical issues for this unique patient population. Appropriate psychiatric screening and management of these patients is believed to play an important role in successful postoperative outcomes.

Jeffrey L. Sebastian

Bariatric surgery remains the treatment of choice for the extremely obese patient, with an exponential growth in the number of procedures performed in response to the obesity epidemic. There are a variety of bariatric procedures available, which differ according to the method in which they achieve sustained weight loss. Plastic surgeons are beginning to see large numbers of patients who have undergone bariatric surgery and who have sustained massive weight loss (MWL) for evaluation of complex and lengthy-body contouring procedures. Proper evaluation of the patient who has sustained MWL requires an understanding of the physiologic impact of different bariatric procedures with particular knowledge of potential long-term nutritional complications.

Editorial Commentary 105

Upper Body Lift 107

Shehab Soliman, Silvia Cristina Rotemberg, Daniele Pace, Adel Bark, Alexander Mansur, Albert Cram, and Al Aly

An upper body lift is needed whenever a massive weight loss patient presents with a "dropped out" lateral inframammary crease. It is a combination of a brachioplasty, upper-back resection, and breast reconstruction. The operation is designed to reverse the particular deformity a patient presents with. This article describes three patterns of resection, one for males and two for females.

Lateral Thoracic Excisions in the Post Massive Weight Loss Patient 115

Susan E. Downey and John E. Gross

The lateral vertical thoracic excision has been a useful adjunct to more traditional techniques. As more patients undergo massive weight loss, more patients will present to plastic surgeons with complaints of fullness and excess in areas of the body not addressed by more traditional techniques. The lateral vertical thoracic excision can offer a solution to a difficult problem.

Editorial Commentary 121

Mastopexy After Massive Weight Loss: Dermal Suspension and Selective Auto-Augmentation 123

J. Peter Rubin and Gerald Khachi

The technique that we outline is extremely versatile for restoring an aesthetic and youthful breast shape in the patient who has lost a massive amount of weight. Overall, complication rates have been low. Despite the disadvantages of a lengthy scar and the need for extensive intraoperative tailoring (which may increase operative time), this operation carries an extremely high rate of patient satisfaction.

L Brachioplasty Correction of Excess Tissue of the Upper Arm, Axilla, and Lateral Chest 131

Dennis J. Hurwitz and Tim Neavin

Following massive weight loss, patients evolve severe arm deformity, extending through the axilla and on to the chest. The L brachioplasty was developed to treat the entire deformity through the excision of two unequal ellipses at right angles in the form of an "L." More than 50 patients have been treated since 2002 with esthetic reshaping of the upper arm, leaving inconspicuous scars and only minor complications. There have been eight scar revisions, including two Z-plasties for contracture. The rationale and results compare favorably with contemporary techniques. L brachioplasty is our procedure of choice for the patient who has had massive weight loss, and it can be applied selectively to the aging arm.

ELSEVIER
SAUNDERS

CLINICS IN
PLASTIC
SURGERY

Clin Plastic Surg 35 (2008) xi–xii

Preface

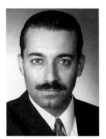

Al Aly, MD, FACS
Iowa City Plastic Surgery
501 12th Avenue, Suite 102
Coralville, IA 52241, USA

E-mail address:
mdplastic@aol.com

Al Aly, MD, FACS
Guest Editor

I was fortunate enough to begin my career in plastic surgery at the University of Iowa, the birthplace of bariatric surgery. Although at the time of my arrival there bariatric surgery had not developed to its present capabilities, Iowa had an abundance of patients who had undergone massive weight loss who provided fertile ground to develop an interest in body contouring. I owe these patients a great deal because they taught me many things that I will always carry with me. I would like to share some of them:

1. Patients who have undergone massive weight loss have worked very hard to lose weight.
2. They are disappointed with their resultant body contour.
3. Their deformities are more severe and intrinsically different from patients who have not undergone massive weight loss.
4. Traditional body contouring techniques, such as abdominoplasty or "T" brachioplasty, are often inadequate in the treatment of these patients.
5. It is our job as plastic surgeons to eliminate the physical stigmata of being "fat." Anything short of that should be a disappointment.
6. Improving body contour does not automatically eliminate psychologic issues.

Since the year 2000, body contouring after massive weight loss has become a subspecialty of plastic surgery that may indeed become the largest subspecialty within the realm of plastic surgery. It is a bona fide subspecialty unto itself because it encompasses a large number of anatomic regions, techniques, and concepts that are unique.

In this issue of the *Clinics in Plastic Surgery* I have asked the authors to provide information on a wide variety of subjects not directly related to surgical technique but essential to what a plastic surgeon should know about bariatric surgery and the appropriate workup of a patient who has undergone massive weight loss. The psychiatric problems of the obese and those who have undergone massive weight loss are also discussed. For each anatomic area that a patient might complain about, a couple of surgical treatment techniques are presented to give the reader a range of differing approaches. It would be impossible to cover all techniques that are available, but I believe the contents of this issue should give the reader a sense

doi:10.1016/j.cps.2007.10.014

of the important concepts. Last, but not least, safety and prevention of complications are discussed.

I have also added some Editorial Commentaries throughout the issue. By their nature these comments are my personal opinions and are based on my experience in this field. They are not meant to encourage or discourage the reader from adopting or discarding the discussed techniques. The reader should evaluate these commentaries critically, as they should the entire issue.

It has been an honor and a privilege to edit this issue of the *Clinics in Plastic Surgery*. I thank all the authors for their hard work and excellent articles. As always, I give special thanks to my teachers and my partner Albert Cram, without whom I cannot do any of this work.

ELSEVIER
SAUNDERS

CLINICS IN
PLASTIC
SURGERY

Clin Plastic Surg 35 (2008) 1–10

Psychiatric Considerations of the Massive Weight Loss Patient

David B. Sarwer, PhD[a,b,*], Anthony N. Fabricatore, PhD[a]

- Preoperative psychiatric functioning of candidates for bariatric surgery
- Does preoperative psychological functioning predict postoperative outcomes?
- Postoperative psychological functioning of patients who undergo bariatric surgery
- Psychological aspects of plastic surgery
- Psychological aspects of body contouring following massive weight loss
- References

Obesity, defined by a body mass index (BMI) of at least 30 kg/m^2, has been identified by the World Health Organization as a "global epidemic" [1]. This problem is especially prominent in the United States, where the prevalence of obesity more than doubled from 15% of adults in 1976–1980 to 32% in 2003–2004 [2,3]. Extreme obesity, characterized by a BMI of at least 40 kg/m^2, has increased even more rapidly, as evidenced by a fourfold increase in prevalence from 1986 to 2000 [4]. Given the effects of excess body weight on cardiovascular, respiratory, and endocrine function, it is no wonder that obesity is considered by many to be one of the most pressing issues in public health [5].

Several studies found that modest weight reductions, of 5% to 10% in initial weight, are associated with significant health benefits for overweight (BMI 25–29.9 kg/m^2) and obese individuals [5]. For persons with extreme obesity, however, more drastic weight losses may be necessary to reduce morbidity

and mortality risks significantly. Furthermore, many extremely obese persons suffer from impairments in quality of life and other psychosocial distress [6–9]. Such disturbances may motivate patients' decisions to seek bariatric surgery, which is the riskiest weight loss method and the most efficacious [5].

The popularity of bariatric surgery has surged in recent years. Whereas 13,365 bariatric procedures were performed in 1998, an estimated 103,000 such surgeries were performed in 2003 [10]. Presently, the most common bariatric procedure in the United States is the Roux-en-y gastric bypass surgery [11]. Adjustable gastric banding (referred to as the LapBand procedure) is gaining popularity in the United States [12]. A meta-analysis found mean reductions of 41.5 kg and 34.8 kg with the gastric bypass and adjustable gastric banding procedures, respectively [13].

There is significant patient-to-patient variability, however, in the long-term results of bariatric

Work on this paper was supported, in part, by the National Institute of Diabetes and Digestive and Kidney Diseases (Grants R03-DK067885 and R01-DK 072452 to Dr. Sarwer and K23-DK070777 to Dr Fabricatore).
[a] Department of Psychiatry, Center for Weight and Eating Disorders, University of Pennsylvania School of Medicine, Philadelphia, PA, USA
[b] Division of Plastic Surgery, Department of Surgery, The Edwin and Fannie Gray Hall Center for Human Appearance, University of Pennsylvania School of Medicine, Philadelphia, PA, USA
* Corresponding author. The Edwin and Fannie Gray Hall Center for Human Appearance, University of Pennsylvania School of Medicine, 10 Penn Tower, 3400 Spruce Street, Philadelphia, PA 19104.
E-mail address: dsarwer@mail.med.upenn.edu (D.B. Sarwer).

doi:10.1016/j.cps.2007.08.006

surgery. One large study, for example, found that 9% of patients who underwent gastric bypass and 25% of patients who underwent adjustable gastric banding had failed to maintain at least a 5% reduction in initial weight 10 years postoperatively [14]. The role of psychological or dietary factors in these suboptimal outcomes is not well understood.

This article reviews psychosocial considerations in patients who seek and receive bariatric surgery. We address preoperative psychological and behavioral characteristics of candidates for bariatric surgery and how those characteristics affect, and are affected by, postoperative weight loss. Because changes in physical appearance are an obvious outcome of bariatric surgery, we review research on the relationship between weight and body image. Many patients seek plastic surgical procedures following massive weight loss. Thus, we review psychological issues related to body-contouring surgery following massive weight loss and discuss the psychological assessment and management of these patients.

Preoperative psychiatric functioning of candidates for bariatric surgery

The significant health problems that are associated with extreme obesity likely motivate many individuals to pursue bariatric surgery. Many extremely obese persons also pursue bariatric surgery for its anticipated effects on their psychosocial status. In the past several years, several comprehensive reviews of the literature on the psychosocial and behavioral aspects of bariatric surgery have been published [6–9,15–18]. This literature is used to inform the summary below.

Numerous studies found a high rate of psychopathology among persons with extreme obesity who pursue bariatric surgery. Between 20% and 60% of patients have been characterized as suffering from an Axis I psychiatric disorder, the most common of which were mood and anxiety disorders [19,20]. Smaller percentages have been diagnosed with substance abuse problems and personality disorders, both of which may impact surgical management and postoperative outcomes [6–9,15–18].

Of these disorders, depression may be the most significant. In a population-based study of more than 40,000 adults in the United States, the risk for major depression in persons with a BMI of at least 40 kg/m² was nearly five times that in persons of average weight (BMI 18.5–24.9 kg/m²) [21]. The risk for depression among patients seeking bariatric surgery may be even greater, because medical and surgical patients typically report more depression than do nontreatment-seeking individuals [22].

Extreme obesity also is associated with reduced health-related quality of life [23–31]. This is not surprising, because extremely obese individuals frequently report significant pain in weight-bearing joints, as well as impaired flexibility and stamina [32–35]. These physical problems lead to difficulties in performing basic activities, such as walking, climbing stairs, bathing, and dressing, which are among the most distressing aspects of extreme obesity [36].

Impairments in quality of life may contribute to the increased risk for depression that is found in persons with extreme obesity. A cross-sectional investigation of quality of life and mood in a sample of patients who underwent bariatric surgery found mean depression scores in the subclinical range for persons with unimpaired physical function, but in the clinically significant range for those whose weight limited their function [24]. This was true in persons with BMIs greater than 60 kg/m², as well as in more typical candidates for bariatric surgery, whose BMIs were in the 40s or 50s.

An important aspect of quality of life is body image. Dissatisfaction with one's body image is believed to motivate many behaviors, including weight loss, exercise, cosmetic and fashion purchases, and cosmetic surgery [37–43]. Overweight and obese individuals, especially women, tend to be more dissatisfied with their bodies and outward appearance than are their normal weight counterparts [40–42,44]. The positive relationship between BMI and body image dissatisfaction may even be stronger than the research suggests, given that many studies did not include persons with extreme obesity [45–52]. Body image dissatisfaction is related to lower self-esteem and increased symptoms of depression in obese individuals, and, therefore is believed to be a marker for other psychological or psychiatric problems [49,51,53–55].

Several studies have focused on the eating behavior of individuals who present for bariatric surgery. The most common and likely relevant condition is binge eating disorder (BED), which is characterized by eating a large amount of food within a 2-hour period of time while feeling a subjective loss of control [56]. (Purging or other compensatory behaviors that are seen in bulimia nervosa are not found in BED.) Although early studies suggested that up to half of candidates for bariatric surgery displayed features of BED [57,58], a recent study, which rigorously applied the diagnostic criteria, suggested that the rate of the disorder may be as low as 5% [59]. Thus, it is clear that this pattern of eating is an anomaly, even among those who are 100 lbs or more overweight. When BED is present, it can be considered a marker for additional psychopathology, because the prevalence of mood, anxiety, personality, and substance-use disorders is greater among persons with this disorder [60,61].

Another factor that may contribute to psychosocial distress in those with extreme obesity is weight-related stigma. Bias against obese individuals has been found in social, educational, occupational, and medical settings and may be associated with discriminatory treatment [62,63]. Although empiric studies have not examined this issue, it is likely that persons with severe obesity experience more pervasive and intense stigma than do their less obese counterparts.

In summary, studies have found high rates of psychopathology, impairments in quality of life, and disordered eating among candidates for bariatric surgery. Results from the investigations of psychopathology and disordered eating, however, must be viewed with caution because of a variety of methodological issues. These limitations have made it difficult to make conclusive statements about the impact of preoperative psychiatric status and eating behavior on postoperative outcome, which is the most important question yet to be addressed definitively by this literature.

Does preoperative psychological functioning predict postoperative outcomes?

Most bariatric surgery programs in the United States require a mental health evaluation as part of the patient selection process [64]. Such evaluations were recommended universally in a 1991 National Institutes of Health consensus development panel statement and recommended on an as-needed basis in a more recent statement by the American Society for Metabolic and Bariatric Surgery [65,66]. Although there is a great deal of variability in the way that preoperative mental health evaluations are conducted, most psychologists and other professionals who perform these assessments agree that significant psychiatric issues contraindicate bariatric surgery [64,67]. Typically cited contraindications include active substance abuse, active psychosis, bulimia nervosa, and severe uncontrolled depression [66,68]. These features are believed to limit the capacity for informed consent or to increase the likelihood of postoperative medical complications.

Whether these and other psychological factors are related to postoperative weight loss is an issue that has not been resolved adequately. There is no clear relationship between preoperative depression and postoperative weight loss. Some studies found that depression was related to less weight loss [69], whereas others found no relationship [53,70,71]. Still others found greater weight loss among persons with more depressive symptoms [72].

Research on the relationship between preoperative binge eating and postoperative weight loss is similarly unclear. Several studies found that the presence of BED predicted suboptimal surgical weight loss or premature weight regain [73,74], but at least one study found no relationship between BED and postoperative outcomes [75]. Many of these investigations, unfortunately, have been limited by several methodological concerns; however, given the potential association with premature weight regain, most programs evaluate for the presence of disordered eating before bariatric surgery [64,67].

In their review of the psychosocial literature, Herpertz and colleagues [7] drew a thought-provoking conclusion. They suggested that psychosocial distress that is secondary to obesity, such as significant body image dissatisfaction or "weight-related" depression, may facilitate weight loss following surgery. In contrast, the presence of significant psychopathology that is independent from the degree of obesity, such as major depression, may inhibit a patient's ability to make the necessary dietary and behavioral changes to have the most successful postoperative outcome possible.

During the prebariatric surgery psychological evaluation, when a formal psychiatric disorder or significant psychological distress is observed, psychiatric or psychological treatment typically is recommended before surgery [76]. This recommendation is typically made to between 25% and 35% of candidates for bariatric surgery [19,67,77]. Of primary concern is ensuring that the distress, whether "garden variety" depression or psychosis, is controlled optimally before exposing patients to the physical discomfort and stress of drastic lifestyle change associated with surgery.

Postoperative psychological functioning of patients who undergo bariatric surgery

The massive weight loss following bariatric surgery is associated with significant improvements in many obesity-related comorbidities [13,78]. Numerous studies found that patients similarly experience improvements in psychosocial status postoperatively [47,70,73,79–88]. As summarized in the comprehensive reviews, most psychosocial characteristics, including self-esteem, depressive symptoms, and health-related quality of life and body image, improve dramatically in the first year after surgery [6–9,15–17]; however, these psychosocial benefits seem to be limited to the first few postoperative years. A growing body of evidence suggests that the occurrence of postoperative binge eating is associated with weight regain within the first 2 years after surgery [57,74,89]. This finding may be particularly important when the timing of body contouring procedures is considered (see later discussion).

Body image may be the most important psychological issue for the patient who has lost a massive amount of weight and is interested in body contouring. Typically, patients who have undergone bariatric surgery report improvements in body image postoperatively. Obese women report improvements in body image following weight loss with behaviorally based programs and bariatric surgery [47,90–92]; however, most studies only investigated changes in the first or, occasionally, second postoperative year. Furthermore, some patients who have undergone bariatric surgery report residual body image dissatisfaction associated with loose, sagging skin of the breasts, abdomen, thighs, and arms following massive weight loss [42]. More than two thirds of patients who have undergone bariatric surgery considered the development of excess skin to be a negative consequence of surgery [93]. This dissatisfaction likely motivates some individuals to seek body-contouring procedures to address these concerns.

Psychological aspects of plastic surgery

Over the past 50 years, a sizable literature has investigated the psychological characteristics of individuals who seek plastic surgery as well as the changes in a range of psychosocial domains postoperatively. As reviewed in detail elsewhere [94], early studies suggested that patients who underwent cosmetic surgery were highly psychopathological. More contemporary investigations found far less psychopathology among those who seek cosmetic surgery. Within the past decade, the focus of this literature has turned to the issues related to body image. Dissatisfaction with one's appearance or body image has long been believed to play a role in an individual's decision to undergo plastic surgery [95–97]. Studies have found repeatedly that patients who undergo cosmetic surgery report heightened body image dissatisfaction before surgery [98–103]. Most patients report significant improvements in their body image postoperatively [104–107]; however, no study has followed patients for more than 2 years postoperatively. As a result, it is unclear if cosmetic surgery leads to longer lasting improvements in body image.

Although heightened body image dissatisfaction seems to be a common characteristic of patients who undergo cosmetic surgery, several studies found that between 7% and 16% of patients meet diagnostic criteria for body dysmorphic disorder (BDD). BDD is characterized by extreme body image dissatisfaction that contributes to a preoccupation with a slight or imagined defect in appearance [100,108–111]. Individuals who have BDD frequently seek plastic surgery and other appearance-enhancing treatments. In contrast to persons who have mild to moderate body image dissatisfaction, most persons who have BDD experience little change or a worsening in their BDD symptoms postoperatively [112,113]. As a result, some authorities consider it a contraindication to plastic surgery [95,114,115]. Because the physical deformities that are found in most patients who have lost a massive amount of weight are neither slight nor imagined, the diagnosis technically cannot be applied to these patients; however, studies of patients undergoing other reconstructive surgical procedures suggest that they often report a level of preoccupation with their appearance that is consistent with BDD [109,111]. Thus, some patients who undergo body contouring likely present for surgery with some form of the disorder, although the exact percentage has yet to be established.

Psychological aspects of body contouring following massive weight loss

As the number of Americans who experience a massive weight loss and present for body-contouring surgery continues to grow, so does our understanding of the surgical treatment of these patients. As in other forms of plastic surgery, understanding the psychological aspects of these patients likely plays an important role in preoperative assessment and postoperative management [116]. The psychosocial and physical outcomes of these procedures, as well as the factors that motivate the decision to seek them, have received little empirical attention [18]. Thus, the larger literature on the psychological aspects of cosmetic surgery, as well as the breast reduction literature, can be used as a framework from which to understand the relevant psychological issues for patients who have lost a massive amount of weight [18,117].

The preoperative psychological assessment of the patient who has lost a massive amount of weight should be a central part of the initial plastic surgery consultation. The assessment should focus on several areas: motivations and expectations, appearance and body image concerns, and psychiatric status and history [18,118–120]. In addition, the plastic surgeon should determine that patients are weight stable at the time of body contouring.

In our current era of "reality-based" cosmetic surgery television, many patients who have lost a massive amount of weight may hold unrealistic expectations about the postoperative results. Some may incorrectly anticipate that body-contouring surgery will result in a total body transformation that makes their bodies comparable to persons who never experienced excessive body weight. Others may not fully understand that body-contouring surgery often produces large and visible scars, skin irregularities, and residual deformities in body shape. Patients should be reminded regularly that although surgery may improve body contour, it will not result in a "perfect" body shape. Patients need to be counseled that multiple, often staged, procedures may be necessary to meet their goals, each of which encompasses further risk, recovery time, and often expense.

The plastic surgeon should inquire about the patient's expectations of the impact that body-contouring surgery will have on romantic and sexual relationships. Surprisingly, at least one study found a higher than anticipated divorce rate following bariatric surgery [121]. It is possible that body-contouring surgery may be associated with similar changes in the dynamics of social and romantic relationships. Patients who express unrealistic expectations (eg, that a troubled marriage may be revived after body contouring) may be more likely to express disappointment and dissatisfaction with their postoperative result, even if the surgeon believes that the result is acceptable.

Patients' subjective perception of the postoperative result is at the heart of the body image concerns of these, and all, plastic surgery procedures. Thus, the assessment of patients' body image is a critical part of the initial consultation. It is useful to have patients describe, in their own words, what they dislike about their appearance. In addition, the degree of dissatisfaction should be assessed. Some body image dissatisfaction is typical among patients who undergo plastic surgery and bariatric surgery. Those who report that they think about their appearance for more than 1 hour each day or those who report that their concerns leads to significant emotional upset or disruption in daily functioning may be experiencing extreme body image dissatisfaction that is suggestive of BDD. These patients likely should undergo a psychological consultation before body-contouring surgery.

The plastic surgeon also should assess the more general psychiatric status and history of patients presenting for body contouring. Approximately 40% of patients who undergo bariatric surgery are engaged in some form of psychiatric treatment [19]. By contrast, approximately 20% of patients who undergo cosmetic surgery and 5% of patients who undergo reconstructive surgery report ongoing psychiatric treatment, most frequently with psychopharmacologic agents [122]. The plastic surgeon is encouraged to contact the treating mental health professional to ensure that body-contouring surgery is appropriate at the present time. Patients who are dissatisfied with their postoperative result

following plastic surgery (including body contouring) have used their preoperative psychiatric history as part of their legal action against the plastic surgeon, arguing that their psychiatric condition prevented them from fully understanding the procedure and its potential outcomes. Written confirmation from the treating mental health professional that the patient is psychiatrically stable may offer some protection to the surgeon in such cases.

Many patients who undergo bariatric surgery receive their psychiatric medications, particularly antidepressant medications, from their primary care physicians [19]; however, the plastic surgeon should not assume that these medications are controlling depressive symptoms appropriately. In these situations, depressive symptoms should be assessed further by the plastic surgeon. Observation of patients' mood, affect, and overall presentation during the body-contouring consultation often provides important clues to the presence of a mood disorder. If one is suspected, neurovegetative symptoms, including sleep, appetite, and concentration, should be assessed. If patients endorse difficulties in any of these areas, they should be asked about the frequency of crying or irritability, social isolation, feelings of hopelessness, and the presence of suicidal thoughts. Affirmative answers to several of these questions necessitate a mental health consultation.

BED may be of particular concern among patients who have lost massive amounts of weight. Recurrence of the behaviors that are characteristic of the disorder have been associated with weight regain 18 to 24 months following bariatric surgery [71,74,82,89]. Even among patients who undergo bariatric surgery and do not have BED, they often regain 5% to 10% of their initial body weight within the first 12 to 36 months after surgery and 10% to 15% over the course of the next decade [14]. Patients who have lost a massive amount of weight often present for body contouring within the first few years after the bariatric procedure. Weight gain following body-contouring surgery may affect postoperative satisfaction and potentially compromise the esthetic result. Thus, the plastic surgeon likely should request that candidates for body contouring remain weight stable for approximately 3 to 6 months before surgery. Weight stability should be confirmed by in-person weigh-ins at the plastic surgeon's office.

We are obviously in the early stages of the growth of body-contouring surgery following massive weight loss. Given the recognized importance of psychosocial factors in bariatric and plastic surgery, it stands to reason that these issues will be equally important in this new area. Unfortunately, there has been little empiric study of these issues. Until such studies are completed, we need to rely on the literature on the psychological aspects of plastic surgery as a framework to organize recommendations on the psychological assessment and management of the patient who has lost a massive amount of weight.

References

[1] World Health Organization. Obesity: preventing and managing the global epidemic. Geneva (IL): World Health Organization; 1998.

[2] Flegal KM, Carroll MD, Ogden CL, et al. Prevalence and trends in obesity among US adults. JAMA 2002;288(14):1723–7.

[3] Ogden CL, Carroll MD, Curtin LR, et al. Prevalence of overweight and obesity in the United States, 1999–2004. JAMA 2006;295(13): 1549–55.

[4] Sturm R. Increases in clinically severe obesity in the United States, 1986-2000. Arch Intern Med 2003;163(18):2146–8.

[5] National Institutes of Health. Clinical guidelines on the identification, evaluation, and treatment of overweight and obesity in adults—the evidence report. Obes Res 1998; 6(Suppl 2):51–209.

[6] Bocchieri LE, Meana M, Fisher BL. A review of psychosocial outcomes of surgery for morbid obesity. J Psychosom Res 2002;52(3):155–65.

[7] Herpertz S, Kielmann R, Wolf AM, et al. Does obesity surgery improve psychosocial functioning? A systematic review. Int J Obes Relat Metab Disord 2003;27(11):1300–14.

[8] van Hout GC, van Oudheusden I, van Heck GL. Psychological profile of the morbidly obese. Obes Surg 2004;14(5):479–88.

[9] Sarwer DB, Wadden TA, Fabricatore AN. Psychosocial and behavioral aspects of bariatric surgery. Obes Res 2005;13(4):639–48.

[10] Santry HP, Gillen DL, Lauderdale DS. Trends in bariatric surgical procedures. JAMA 2005; 294(15):1909–17.

[11] Nguyen NT, Root J, Zainabadi K, et al. Accelerated growth of bariatric surgery with the introduction of minimally invasive surgery. Arch Surg 2005;140(12):1198–202.

[12] Buchwald H, Williams SE. Bariatric surgery worldwide 2003. Obes Surg 2004;14(9): 1157–64.

[13] Maggard MA, Shugarman LR, Suttorp M, et al. Meta-analysis: surgical treatment of obesity. Ann Intern Med 2005;142(7):547–9.

[14] Sjostrom L, Lindroos AK, Peltonen M, et al. Lifestyle, diabetes, and cardiovascular risk factors 10 years after bariatric surgery. N Engl J Med 2004;351(26):2683–93.

[15] Herpertz S, Kielmann R, Wolf AM, et al. Do psychosocial variables predict weight loss or mental health after obesity surgery? A systematic review. Obes Res 2004;12(10):1554–69.

[16] Mitchell JE, de Zwaan M. Bariatric surgery: a guide for mental health professionals. New York: Routledge; 2005.

[17] van Hout GC, Boekestein P, Fortuin FA, et al. Psychosocial functioning following bariatric surgery. Obes Surg 2006;16(6):787–94.

[18] Sarwer DB, Thompson JK, Mitchell JE. Psychological considerations of the bariatric surgery patient interested in body contouring surgery. Plast Reconstr Surg, in press.

[19] Sarwer DB, Cohn NI, Gibbons LM, et al. Psychiatric diagnoses and psychiatric treatment among bariatric surgery candidates. Obes Surg 2004;14(9):1148–56.

[20] Rosenberger PR, Henderson KE, Grilo CM. Psychiatric disorder comorbidity and association with eating disorders in bariatric surgery patients: a cross-sectional study using structured interview-based diagnosis. J Clin Psychiatry 2006;67(7):1080–5.

[21] Onyike CU, Crum RM, Lee HB, et al. Is obesity associated with major depression? Results from the Third National Health and Nutrition Examination Survey. Am J Epidemiol 2003;158(12): 1139–47.

[22] Swenson WM, Pearson JS, Osborne D. An MMPI source book: basic item, scale and pattern data on 50,000 medical patients. Minneapolis (MN): University of Minnesota Press; 1973.

[23] Choban PS, Onyejekwe J, Burge JC, et al. A health status assessment of the impact of weight loss following Roux-en-Y gastric bypass for clinically severe obesity. J Am Coll Surg 1999;188(5):491–7.

[24] Fabricatore AN, Wadden TA, Sarwer DB, et al. Health-related quality of life and symptoms of depression in extremely obese persons seeking bariatric surgery. Obes Surg 2005;15(3): 304–9.

[25] Fontaine KR, Cheskin LJ, Barofsky I. Health-related quality of life in obese persons seeking treatment. J Fam Pract 1996;43(3): 265–720.

[26] Kolotkin RL, Crosby RD, Pendleton R, et al. Health-related quality of life in patients seeking gastric bypass surgery vs non-treatment-seeking controls. Obes Surg 2003;13(3):371–7.

[27] Kolotkin RL, Crosby RD, Williams GR. Health-related quality of life varies among obese subgroups. Obes Res 2002;10(8):748–56.

[28] Kolotkin RL, Crosby RD, Williams GR, et al. The relationship between health-related quality of life and weight loss. Obes Res 2001;9(9): 564–71.

[29] Schok M, Greenen R, van Antwerpen T, et al. Quality of life after laparoscopic adjustable gastric banding for severe obesity: postoperative and retrospective preoperative evaluations. Obes Surg 2000;10(6):502–8.

[30] Larsson U, Karlsson J, Sullivan M. Impact of overweight and obesity on health-related quality of life - a Swedish population study. Int J Obes Relat Metab Disord 2002;26(3): 417–24.

[31] Mathus-Vliegen EM, deWeerd S, de Wit LT. Health related quality-of-life in patients with morbid obesity after gastric banding for surgically induced weight loss. Surgery 2004; 135(5):489–97.

[32] Larsson UE, Mattsson E. Functional limitations linked to high body mass index, age and current pain in obese women. Int J Obes 2001; 25(6):893–9.

[33] Larsson UE, Mattsson E. Perceived disability and observed functional limitations in obese women. Int J Obes Relat Metab Disord 2001; 25(11):1705–12.

[34] Peltonen M, Lindroos AK, Torgerson JS. Musculoskeletal pain in the obese: a comparison with a general population and long-term changes after conventional and surgical obesity treatment. Pain 2003;104(3):549–57.

[35] Karason K, Peltonen M, Lindroos AK, et al. Effort-related calf pain in the obese and long-term changes after surgical obesity treatment. Obes Res 2005;13(1):137–45.

[36] Duval K, Marceau P, Lescelleur O, et al. Health-related quality of life in morbid obesity. Obes Surg 2006;16(5):574–9.

[37] Cash TF. A "negative body image": evaluating epidemiological evidence. In: Cash TF, Pruzinsky T, editors. Body image: a handbook of theory, research & clinical practice. New York: Guilford Press; 2004. p. 269–76.

[38] Sarwer DB, Didie ER. Body image in cosmetic surgical and dermatological practice. In: Castle D, Phillips KA, editors. Disorders of body image. Stroud (UK): Wrighton Biomedical Publishing; 2002. p. 37–53.

[39] Sarwer DB, Allison KC, Berkowitz RI. Assessment and treatment of obesity in the primary care setting. In: Hass LJ, editor. Handbook of primary-care psychology. New York: Oxford University Press; 2004. p. 435–54.

[40] Sarwer DB, Foster GD, Wadden TA. Treatment of obesity I: adult obesity. In: Thompson JK, editor. Handbook of eating disorders and obesity. Hoboken (NJ): Wiley; 2004. p. 421–42.

[41] Sarwer DB, Thompson JK. Obesity and body image disturbance. In: Wadden TA, Stunkard AJ, editors. Handbook of obesity treatment. New York: Guilford Press; 2002. p. 447–64.

[42] Sarwer DB, Thompson JK, Cash TF. Body image and obesity in adulthood. Psychiatr Clin North Am 2005;28(1):69–87.

[43] Sarwer DB, Magee L. Physical appearance and society. In: Sarwer DB, Pruzinsky T, Cash TF, et al, editors. Psychological aspects of reconstructive and cosmetic plastic surgery: clinical, empirical, and ethical perspectives.

Philadelphia: Lippincott, Williams, Wilkins; 2006. p. 23–36.

[44] Schwartz MB, Brownell KD. Obesity and body image. Body Image 2004;1(1):43–56.

[45] Hill AJ, Williams J. Psychological heath in a non-clinical sample of obese women. Int J Obes Relat Metab Disord 1998;22(6):578–83.

[46] Sarwer DB, Gibbons LM, Wadden TA. The relationship between body mass and body image dissatisfaction. Presented at the North American Association for the Study of Obesity Annual Meeting. Las Vegas. November 14–18, 2004.

[47] Dixon JB, Dixon ME, O'Brien PE. Body image: appearance orientation and evaluation in the severely obese. Changes with weight loss. Obes Surg 2002;12(1):65–71.

[48] Eldrige KL, Agras WS. Weight and shape overconcern and emotional eating in binge eating disorder. Int J Eat Disord 1996;19(1):73–82.

[49] Foster GD, Wadden TA, Vogt RA. Body image in obese women before, during, and after weight loss treatment. Health Psychol 1997;16(3):226–9.

[50] Matz PE, Foster GD, Faith MS, et al. Correlates of body image dissatisfaction among overweight women seeking weight loss. J Consult Clin Psychol 2002;70(4):1040–4.

[51] Sarwer DB, Wadden TA, Foster GD. Assessment of body image dissatisfaction in obese women: specificity, severity, and clinical significance. J Consult Clin Psychol 1998;66(4):651–4.

[52] Wilfley DE, Schreiber GB, Pike KM, et al. Eating disturbance and body image: a comparison of a community sample of adult black and white women. Int J Eat Disord 1996;20(4):377–87.

[53] Dixon JB, Dixon ME, O'Brien PE. Pre-operative predictors of weight loss at 1-year after the Lap-Band surgery. Obes Surg 2001;11(2):200–7.

[54] Grilo CM, Wilfley DE, Brownell KD, et al. Teasing, body image, and self-esteem in a clinical sample of obese women. Addict Behav 1994; 19(4):443–50.

[55] Neumark-Sztainer D, Haines J. Psychosocial and behavioral consequences of obesity. In: Thompson JK, editor. Handbook of eating disorders and obesity. Hoboken (NJ): Wiley; 2004. p. 349–71.

[56] American Psychiatric Association. Diagnostic and statistical manual of mental disorders. 4th edition, Text Revision. Washington, DC: APA Press; 2000.

[57] Mitchell JE, Lancaster KL, Burgard MA, et al. Long-term follow-up of patients' status after gastric bypass. Obes Surg 2001;11(4):464–78.

[58] Wadden TA, Sarwer DB, Arnold ME, et al. Psychosocial status of severely obese patients before and after bariatric surgery. Problems in General Surgery 2000;17:13–22.

[59] Allison KC, Thomas WA, Sarwer DB, et al. Night eating syndrome and binge eating disorder among persons seeking bariatric surgery: prevalence and related features. Surg Obes Relat Dis 2006;2(2):153–8.

[60] Stunkard AJ, Allison KC. Binge eating disorder: disorder or marker? Int J Eat Disord 2003; 34(Suppl):S107–16.

[61] Allison KC, Stunkard AJ. Obesity and eating disorders. Psychiatr Clin North Am 2005;28(1): 55–67.

[62] Puhl RM, Brownell KD. Bias, discrimination, and obesity. Obes Res 2001;9(12):788–805.

[63] Brownell KD, Puhl RM, Schwartz MB, et al. Weight bias: nature, consequences, and remedies. New York: Guilford Press; 2005.

[64] Bauchowitz AU, Gonder-Frederick LA, Olbrisch ME, et al. Psychosocial evaluation of bariatric surgery candidates: a survey of present practices. Psychosom Med 2005;67(5):825–32.

[65] Hubbard VS, Hall WH. Gastrointestinal surgery for severe obesity. Obes Surg 1991;1(3):257–65.

[66] Buchwald H. Bariatric surgery for morbid obesity: health implications for patients, health professionals, and third-party payers. J Am Coll Surg 2005;200(4):593–604.

[67] Fabricatore AN, Crerand CE, Wadden TA, et al. How do mental health professionals evaluate candidates for bariatric surgery? Survey results. Obes Surg 2006;16(5):567–73.

[68] Wadden TA, Sarwer DB, Womble LG, et al. Psychosocial aspects of obesity and obesity surgery. Surg Clin North Am 2001;81(5):1001–24.

[69] Kinzl JF, Schrattenecker M, Traweger C, et al. Psychosocial predictors of weight loss after bariatric surgery. Obes Surg 2006;16(12):1609–14.

[70] Powers PS, Rosemurgy A, Boyd F, et al. Outcome of gastric restriction procedures: weight, psychiatric diagnoses, and satisfaction. Obes Surg 1997;7(6):471–7.

[71] Hsu LK, Benotti PN, Dwyer J, et al. Nonsurgical factors that influence the outcome of bariatric surgery: a review. Psychosom Med 1998;60(3): 338–46.

[72] Averbukh Y, Heshka S, El-Shoreya H, et al. Depression score predicts weight loss following Roux-en-Y gastric bypass. Obes Surg 2003; 13(6):833–6.

[73] Dymek MP, le Grange D, Neven K, et al. Quality of life and psychosocial adjustment in patients after Roux-en-Y gastric bypass: a brief report. Obes Surg 2001;11(1):32–9.

[74] Kalarchian MA, Marcus MD, Wilson GT, et al. Binge eating among gastric bypass patients at long-term follow-up. Obes Surg 2002;12(2): 270–5.

[75] White MA, Masheb RM, Rothschild BS, et al. The prognostic significance of regular binge eating in extremely obese gastric bypass patients: 12-month postoperative outcomes. J Clin Psychiatry 2006;67(12):1928–35.

[76] Wadden TA, Sarwer DB, Fabricatore AN, et al. Psychosocial and behavioral status of bariatric surgery patients: what to expect before and after surgery. Med Clin North Am 2007;91:451–69.

[77] Pawlow LA, O'Neil PM, White MA, et al. Findings and outcomes of psychological evaluations of gastric bypass applicants. Surg Obes Relat Dis 2005;1(6):523–7.

[78] Buchwald H, Avidor Y, Braunwald E, et al. Bariatric surgery: a systematic review and meta-analysis. JAMA 2004;292(14):1724–37.

[79] Adami GF, Gandolfo P, Campostano A, et al. Eating disorder inventory in the assessment of psychosocial status in the obese patients prior to and at long-term following biliopancreatic diversion for obesity. Int J Eat Disord 1994; 15(3):265–74.

[80] Dixon JB, Dixon ME, O'Brien PE. Depression in association with severe obesity: changes with weight loss. Arch Intern Med 2003;163(17): 2058–65.

[81] Gentry K, Halverson JD, Heisler S. Psychologic assessment of morbidly obese patients undergoing gastric bypass: a comparison of preoperative and postoperative adjustment. Surgery 1984; 95(2):215–20.

[82] Karlsson J, Sjostrom L, Sullivan M. Swedish obese subjects (SOS)—an intervention study of obesity. Two-year follow-up of health-related quality of life (HRQL) and eating behavior after gastric surgery for severe obesity. Int J Obes Relat Metab Disord 1998;22(2):113–26.

[83] Maddi SR, Fox SR, Khoshaba DM, et al. Reduction in psychopathology following bariatric surgery for morbid obesity. Obes Surg 2001; 11(6):680–5.

[84] Malone M, Alger-Mayer S. Binge status and quality of life after gastric bypass surgery: a one-year study. Obes Res 2004;12(3):473–81.

[85] Solow C, Silberfarb PM, Swift K. Psychosocial effects of intestinal bypass surgery for severe obesity. N Engl J Med 1974;290(6):300–4.

[86] Vallis TM, Butler GS, Perey B, et al. The role of psychological functioning in morbid obesity and its treatment with gastroplasty. Obes Surg 2001;11(6):716–25.

[87] van Gemert WG, Adang EM, Greve JW, et al. Quality of life assessment of morbidly obese patients: effect of weight-reducing surgery. Am J Clin Nutr 1998;67(2):197–201.

[88] Waters GS, Pories WJ, Swanson MS, et al. Long-term studies of mental health after the Greenville gastric bypass operation for morbid obesity. Am J Surg 1991;161(1):154–7.

[89] Kalarchian MA, Wilson GT, Brolin RE, et al. Effects of bariatric surgery on binge eating and related psychopathology. Eat Weight Disord 1999;4(1):1–5.

[90] Adami GF, Gandolfo P, Campostano A, et al. Body image and body weight in obese patients. Int J Eat Disord 1998;24(3):299–306.

[91] Camps MA, Zervos E, Goode S, et al. Impact of bariatric surgery on body image perception and sexuality in morbidly obese patients and their partners. Obes Res 1996;6(4):356–60.

[92] Neven K, Dymek M, le Grange D, et al. The effects of Roux-en-Y gastric bypass surgery on body image. Obes Surg 2002;12(2):265–9.

[93] Kinzl JF, Traweger C, Trefalt E, et al. Psychosocial consequences of weight loss following gastric banding for morbid obesity. Obes Surg 2003;13(1):105–10.

[94] Sarwer DB, Didie ER, Gibbons LM. Cosmetic surgery of the body. In: Sarwer DB, Pruzinsky T, Cash TF, et al, editors. Psychological aspects of reconstructive and cosmetic plastic surgery: clinical, empirical, and ethical perspectives. Philadelphia: Lippincott, Williams, Wilkins; 2006. p. 251–66.

[95] Sarwer DB, Crerand CE. Body image and cosmetic medical treatments. Body Image 2004; 1(1):99–111.

[96] Sarwer DB, Wadden TA, Pertschuk MJ, et al. The psychology of cosmetic surgery: a review and reconceptualization. Clin Psychol Rev 1998; 18(1):1–22.

[97] Cash TF. Body image and cosmetic surgery. In: Sarwer DB, Pruzinsky T, Cash TF, et al, editors. Psychological aspects of reconstructive and cosmetic plastic surgery: clinical, empirical, and ethical perspectives. Philadelphia: Lippincott, Williams, Wilkins; 2006. p. 37–59.

[98] Pertschuk MJ, Sarwer DB, Wadden TA, et al. Body image dissatisfaction in male cosmetic surgery patients. Aesthetic Plast Surg 1998; 22(1):20–4.

[99] Sarwer DB, Bartlett SP, Bucky LP, et al. Bigger is not always better: body image dissatisfaction in breast reduction and breast augmentation patients. Plast Reconstr Surg 1998;101(7): 1956–61.

[100] Sarwer DB, Wadden TA, Pertschuk MJ, et al. Body image dissatisfaction and body dysmorphic disorder in 100 cosmetic surgery patients. Plast Reconstr Surg 1998;101(6): 1644–9.

[101] Sarwer DB, Whitaker LA, Wadden TA, et al. Body image dissatisfaction in women seeking rhytidectomy or blepharoplasty. Aesthetic Surg J 1997;17(4):230–4.

[102] Didie ER, Sarwer DB. Factors that influence the decision to undergo cosmetic breast augmentation surgery. J Womens Health 2003;12(3): 241–53.

[103] Sarwer DB, LaRossa D, Bartlett SP, et al. Body image concerns of breast augmentation patients. Plast Reconstr Surg 2003;112(1): 83–90.

[104] Bolton MA, Pruzinsky T, Cash TF, et al. Measuring outcomes in plastic surgery: body image and quality of life in abdominoplasty patients. Plast Reconstr Surg 2003;112(2):619–25.

[105] Cash TF, Duel LA, Perkins LL. Women's psychosocial outcomes of breast augmentation with silicone gel-filled implants: a 2-year prospective study. Plast Reconstr Surg 2002;109(6): 2112–21.

[106] Sarwer DB, Gibbons LM, Magee L, et al. A prospective, multi-site investigation of patient satisfaction and psychosocial status following cosmetic surgery. Aesthetic Surg J 2005;25(3): 263–9.

[107] Sarwer DB, Wadden TA, Whitaker LA. An investigation of changes in body image following cosmetic surgery. Plast Reconstr Surg 2002; 109(1):363–9.

[108] Aouizerate B, Pujol H, Grabot D, et al. Body dysmorphic disorder in a sample of cosmetic surgery applicants. Eur Psychiatry 2003;18(7): 365–8.

[109] Crerand CE, Sarwer DB, Magee L, et al. Rate of body dysmorphic disorder among patients seeking facial plastic surgery. Psychiatr Ann 2004;34:58–965.

[110] Ishigooka J, Iwao M, Suzuki M, et al. Demographic features of patients seeking cosmetic surgery. Psychiatry Clin Neurosci 1998;52(3): 283–7.

[111] Sarwer DB, Whitaker LA, Pertschuk MJ, et al. Body image concerns of reconstructive surgery patients: an underrecognized problem. Ann Plast Surg 1998;40(4):403–7.

[112] Crerand CE, Phillips KA, Menard W, et al. Nonpsychiatric medical treatment of body dysmorphic disorder. Psychosomatics 2005;46(6): 549–55.

[113] Phillips KA, Grant J, Siniscalchi J, et al. Surgical and nonpsychiatric medical treatment of patients with body dysmorphic disorder. Psychosomatics 2001;42(6):504–10.

[114] Crerand CE, Cash TF, Whitaker LA. Cosmetic surgery of the face. In: Sarwer DB, Pruzinsky T, Cash TF, et al, editors. Psychological aspects of reconstructive and cosmetic plastic surgery: clinical, empirical, and ethical perspectives. Philadelphia: Lippincott, Williams, Wilkins; 2006. p. 233–49.

[115] Crerand CE, Franklin ME, Sarwer DB. Body dysmorphic disorder and cosmetic surgery. Plast Reconstr Surg 2006;118(7):167e–89e.

[116] Sarwer DB, Pruzinsky T, Cash TF, et al. Psychological aspects of reconstructive and cosmetic plastic surgery: clinical, empirical, and ethical perspectives. Philadelphia: Lippincott, Williams, Wilkins; 2006.

[117] Young VL, Watson ME. Breast reduction. In: Sarwer DB, Pruzinsky T, Cash TF, et al, editors. Psychological aspects of reconstructive and cosmetic plastic surgery: clinical, empirical, and ethical perspectives. Philadelphia: Lippincott, Williams, Wilkins; 2006. p. 189–206.

[118] Sarwer DB, Grossbat TA, Baker AW. Psychosocial evaluation of the cosmetic surgery patient. In: Kaminer M, Dover J, Arndt K, et al, editors. Atlas of cosmetic surgery. 2nd edition. London: Elsevier; in press.

[119] Sarwer DB. Psychological considerations in cosmetic surgery. In: Goldwyn RM, Cohen MN, editors. The unfavorable result in plastic surgery: avoidance and treatment. 3rd edition. Philadelphia: Lippincott-Raven; 2001. p. 14–23.

[120] Sarwer DB. Psychological assessment of cosmetic surgery patients. In: Sarwer DB, Pruzinsky T, Cash TF, et al, editors. Psychological aspects of reconstructive and cosmetic plastic surgery: clinical, empirical, and ethical perspectives. Philadelphia: Lippincott, Williams, Wilkins; 2006. p. 267–83.

[121] Rand CS, Kuldau JM, Robbins L. Surgery for obesity and marriage quality. JAMA 1982; 247(10):1419–22.

[122] Sarwer DB, Zanville HA, LaRossa D, et al. Mental health histories and psychiatric medication usage among persons who sought cosmetic surgery. Plast Reconstr Surg 2004;114(7):1927–33.

ELSEVIER
SAUNDERS

CLINICS IN
PLASTIC
SURGERY

Clin Plastic Surg 35 (2008) 11–26

Bariatric Surgery and Work-Up of the Massive Weight Loss Patient

Jeffrey L. Sebastian, MD[a,b]

In recent years, plastic surgeons have witnessed an exponential growth in the number of patients presenting for body-contouring procedures following massive weight loss (MWL), which can be defined as 50% or greater loss of excess weight [1], with patients often having lost 100 lbs or more [2]. Although the patient who has sustained MWL is not new to the field of plastic surgery [2–5], the obesity epidemic has resulted in greater numbers seeking evaluation for complex and lengthy body-contouring procedures following bariatric surgery (Fig. 1). The primary goal of the plastic and reconstructive surgeon in operating on the patient who has undergone bariatric surgery and sustained MWL is to provide improvement in form and function in the safest possible setting. Unique to these patients are important considerations that require the plastic surgeon to differentiate the bariatric procedures currently in use, understand the physiologic changes that follow these procedures, and anticipate potential late complications, of which nutritional deficiencies predominate.

The obesity epidemic

In the last 2 decades, there has been a dramatic increase in the prevalence of obesity in the United States and worldwide. In 1995, there were no states with obesity prevalence rates exceeding 20%; in contrast, by 2005, only 4 states had obesity prevalence rates of less than 20%, and 17 states had rates exceeding 25% (Fig. 2) [6]. By current estimates,

[a] David Geffen School of Medicine at UCLA, Los Angeles, CA, USA
[b] Private Practice, Santa Monica, CA, USA
E-mail address: jsebasti@ucla.edu

doi:10.1016/j.cps.2007.08.004

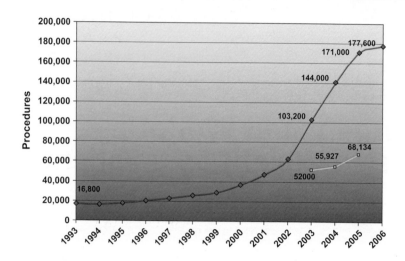

Fig. 1. The growth of bariatric surgery and body-contouring surgery for the massive weight loss patient in the United States. Dark line = bariatric procedures (estimates provided by the American Society for Bariatric Surgery, Gainesville, FL). White line = MWL body-contouring procedures (estimates provided by the American Society of Plastic Surgeons).

approximately 66% of United States adults are overweight or obese, of which 5 million can be classified as extremely obese. Even more alarming has been the dramatic increase in obesity prevalence rates among younger age groups, with 17.1% of children and adolescents currently classified as being overweight [6,7].

Obesity classification

Current definitions of overweight and obesity use the body mass index (BMI) calculation. This is calculated as weight in kilograms divided by the square of height in meters (kg/m^2), with BMI the standard by which to classify weight [8]. The 1998 National Institutes of Health Clinical Guidelines described three classes of overweight and obesity in adults using BMI [9], and the American Society for Bariatric Surgery has expanded terminology to include the most extreme forms of obesity (Fig. 3) [10]. Overweight is defined as a BMI between 25.0 and 29.9 kg/m^2, and extreme or class III obesity is defined as a BMI exceeding 40 kg/m^2.

Obesity health implications

In general, there is a direct correlation between BMI and health implications, although in athletic individuals with a greater proportion of lean body mass, the BMI calculation is less reliable. The health consequences of obesity are numerous and include metabolic complications, cardiovascular disease, respiratory problems, osteoarthritis, and increased risk for a variety of cancers [11,12]. Obesity also seems to be a risk factor for early mortality [13]. The cost of treating obesity and its complications is estimated to exceed $117 billion annually [14].

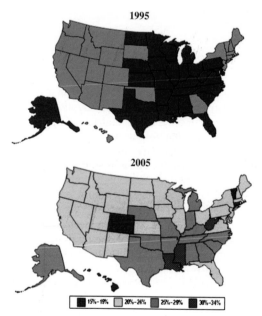

Fig. 2. Maps showing the increasing prevalence of obesity among United States adults (BMI ≥ 30 kg/m^2 or ~30 lbs overweight for a 5′4″ person). (*From* Centers for Disease Control. U.S. Obesity Trends 1985–2006. Available at: http://www.cdc.gov/NCCDPHP/dnpa/obesity/trend/maps/index.htm.)

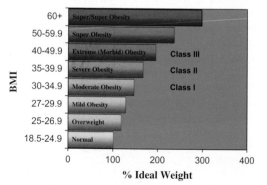

Fig. 3. Obesity classification.

Obesity treatment strategies

In the most basic terms, weight gain or obesity results from an imbalance in energy intake and energy expenditure, resulting in a net positive energy balance. These energy requirements are influenced by several variables, including dietary intake, physical activity, genetics, and certain disease states. The goal in weight management is to produce a net energy deficit resulting in weight loss. There is a greater recognition that obesity is a chronic disease and that any form of treatment aims at palliation rather than cure [15].

Diet

Regulating dietary intake is one of the most important components in the treatment of obesity [16]. Caloric restriction can be achieved by low calorie diets and very low calorie diets. Low calorie diets restrict daily caloric intake by 500 to 1000 kcal per day, with a goal of inducing a 1- to 2-lb weight reduction per week [17]. Very low calorie diets provide 200 to 800 kcal per day and are used often when there is a need to achieve more rapid weight loss, although results do not differ significantly at 1 year [18]. Success ultimately relies on reducing energy intake [19–21], despite considerable controversy regarding the optimum macronutrient composition (eg, low fat versus low carbohydrate) in a diet.

Behavior modification

Behavior therapy aims to modify behavior with regard to energy consumption. Often, it is integral to a comprehensive weight loss program, involving self-monitoring, stimulus control, cognitive behavior modification, goal setting, self-esteem, assertiveness training, relaxation exercises, nutrition, stress management, and social support, among others [22].

Exercise

Physical activity or exercise is important in the treatment of obesity and is a valuable tool in any weight-reduction program. Exercise alone, however, produces only small weight losses [23], with its greatest role apparent in long-term weight loss maintenance [24].

Pharmacotherapy

The US Food and Drug Administration–approved drugs are limited to treating obesity in individuals with BMIs exceeding 30 kg/m^2 or 27 kg/m^2 and greater in the presence of obesity-related disease [17]. Unfortunately, the history of drug therapy for treating obesity is tainted by numerous adverse outcomes, including most recently, the association between valvular heart disease and fenfluramine-phentermine (Fen-Phen) [25]. Current drugs act primarily as appetite suppressants with the exception of orlistat (Xenical), which reduces intestinal digestion and absorption of dietary fat. Only two drugs, orlistat and sibutramine (Meridia), are approved for longer-term (up to 2 years) use [26].

Unfortunately, although modest weight reduction can be achieved through diet, exercise, behavior modification, and drug therapy, evidence suggests that there is a high incidence of relapse, with greater than 90% of individuals regaining weight [27,28].

Bariatric surgery

The most radical option, bariatric surgery, remains the treatment of choice for the severely obese patient who has failed all other methods of weight loss [29]. At least 1 in 20 adults in the United States currently qualifies for bariatric surgery [30]. With the availability of long-term data demonstrating the safety and durability of weight loss with gastric bypass surgery [31,32], there has been an exponential growth in bariatric procedures in the last 5 years (see **Fig. 1**).

Indications for bariatric surgery

The guidelines for selecting candidates for bariatric surgery were put forth by a 1991 National Institutes of Health Consensus Statement (**Box 1**) [33]. Qualified patients typically have a BMI exceeding 40 kg/m^2 or one between 35 and 40 kg/m^2 in the presence of high-risk comorbid conditions. There has been a move to lower BMI requirements to include those with class I obesity in the presence of a comorbid condition that can be improved significantly or cured with substantial weight reduction [34]. There also must be demonstration of failed medical therapy and thorough evaluation by a multidisciplinary team, typically providing medical, surgical, nutritional, and psychiatric expertise. Patients also must be motivated with realistic expectations and committed to long-term follow-up.

Box 1: Requirements for bariatric surgery

BMI$\geq$40 kg/m^2 or BMI 35 to 40 kg/m^2 in the presence of comorbid conditions
Failed medical management
Multidisciplinary evaluation
Motivated, well-informed patient with realistic expectations
Commitment of long-term follow-up

Data from Gastrointestinal Surgery for Severe Obesity. NIH Consensus Statement 1991 Mar 25–27;9(1):1–20.

The evolution of bariatric surgery

Bariatric surgery emerged in the 1950s with observations of MWL in patients with short gut syndrome, leading to the first published report of the jejunoileal bypass (JIB) performed for weight reduction [35]. This was a purely malabsorptive procedure, in which most of the nutrient absorptive surface of the gastrointestinal tract was bypassed by creating an anastomosis from the proximal to the distal small bowel (Fig. 4). The JIB was extremely effective at achieving significant weight loss and enjoyed popularity during the 1960s and 1970s. There were numerous modifications that varied the length of small bowel to be bypassed, as well as a technique that performed direct anastomosis of the proximal small bowel to the colon [36–39]. The most widely adopted procedure was known as the 14″ + 4″ end-to-side jejunoileostomy, in which an anastomosis was created between the proximal 14 inches of jejunum and the terminal ileum, four inches from the ileocecal valve [40]. Although there was tremendous success in achieving weight loss, and despite numerous subsequent modifications, there were severe consequences related to significant and sustained malabsorption of nutrients and bile salt losses in the stool, including electrolyte imbalance, steatorrhea, and nephrolithiasis [41,42]. The most severe of these

was hepatic failure, which eventually led to the abandonment of the JIB; most patients eventually underwent reversal or conversion to another procedure.

Bariatric surgery evolved over the next few decades, with the goal to develop procedures that provided a balance between significant and sustained weight loss and the risk for morbidity and mortality. Innovation led to various surgical procedures that used gastric restriction to limit food intake or procedures that continued to rely heavily upon intestinal malabsorption to achieve weight loss. At the present time, there are three main categories of bariatric procedures: restrictive, malabsorptive, and combination restrictive-malabsorptive.

Restrictive

Surgical stapling devices ushered in the development of purely restrictive procedures in the 1970s and 1980s, including the horizontal gastroplasty [43], gastric partitioning [44], silastic ring gastroplasty [45,46], and the vertical banded gastroplasty(VBG) [47]. These procedures produced satiety by creating a small gastric pouch with a restricted outlet and completely eliminating the undesirable effects seen with alterations in digestion and malabsorption of nutrients from bypassing the gastrointestinal tract. The earliest of these procedures eventually were plagued by weight regain that was due to staple line failures. The most popular of these procedures was the VBG [47], which reinforced the outlet of the pouch with polypropylene mesh, preventing the stoma from stretching (Fig. 5).

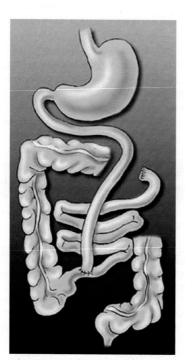

Fig. 4. The jejunoileal bypass. (*Courtesy of* the American Society for Bariatric Surgery, Gainesville, FL; with permission.)

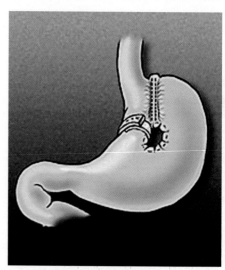

Fig. 5. The vertical banded gastroplasty. (*Courtesy of* the American Society for Bariatric Surgery, Gainesville, FL; with permission.)

The idea of pure restriction was carried one step further with the development of an adjustable silastic gastric band placed around the proximal stomach (Fig. 6) [48]. In 2001, the FDA approved the Bioenterics LAP-BAND System (Allergan, Inc., Irvine, California) (Fig. 7). This band is placed laparoscopically and is considered the least invasive of bariatric procedures. The band diameter can be changed by adjusting a balloon that is connected to a subcutaneously placed access port. The adjustable gastric band has nearly replaced the VBG as a purely restrictive procedure. Outside of the United States, placement of an adjustable gastric band has become the procedure of choice.

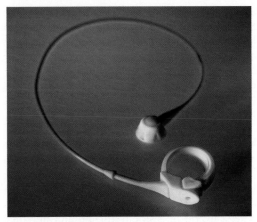

Fig. 7. The Bioenterics LAP-BAND System. (*Courtesy of* Allergan, Irvine, CA.)

Malabsorptive

Recognizing that malabsorption was an effective tool for achieving sustained weight loss, the biliopancreatic diversion (BPD) was developed in the mid 1970s [49]. Unlike the JIB, this procedure incorporates a degree of restriction with a partial gastrectomy, although its primary effectiveness lies with the creation of a short distal common channel where food and digestive enzymes are allowed to mix, leading to malabsorption of nutrients. In contrast to the JIB, the bypassed segment of small bowel, also referred to as the biliopancreatic limb, is maintained in a functional state with the flow of bile and digestive enzymes. This significantly reduces the development of liver cirrhosis from intestinal stasis and bacterial overgrowth.

The duodenal switch (DS) procedure is a modification of the original BPD, in which a sleeve gastrectomy and Roux-en-Y duodenostomy are performed to allow for greater absorption of vitamin B_{12}, as well as a reduction in the incidence of dumping syndrome and stomal ulcer formation (Fig. 8) [50]. Patients often favor the BPD/DS procedure because they do not experience significant restriction with regard to intake and food tolerance, despite

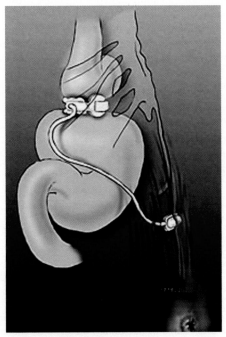

Fig. 6. The adjustable silastic gastric band. (*Courtesy of* the American Society for Bariatric Surgery, Gainesville, FL; with permission.)

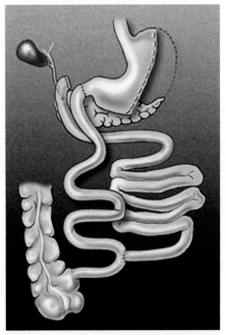

Fig. 8. The biliopancreatic diversion with duodenal switch. (*Courtesy of* the American Society for Bariatric Surgery, Gainesville, FL; with permission.)

achieving rapid and significant weight loss. The BPD, however, does carry the highest risk for long-term nutritional and metabolic complications and often leads to undesirable effects, including frequent loose, foul-smelling stools. Therefore, malabsorptive procedures are in limited use and typically are reserved for superobese patients [51], with BMIs exceeding 50 kg/m².

Combination restrictive-malabsorptive

A different approach to bariatric surgery developed in the 1960s from observations of sustained weight loss following partial gastrectomy for peptic ulcer disease [52]. This led to the gastric bypass procedure, a hybrid of gastric restriction and intestinal malabsorption. Early gastric bypass consisted of a partial gastrectomy, leaving a 100- to 150-mL gastric pouch that was drained with a loop gastroenterostomy [53]. There have been numerous modifications over the last few decades, involving variations in gastric partitioning [54], silastic ring restriction of the gastric pouch [55], reinforcement of the gastrojejunal outlet to avoid enlargement with time, and lengthening of the enteric limb [56]. One major modification has been the creation of a Roux-en-Y anastomosis [57] to reduce the incidence of alkaline gastritis that is due to bile reflux. This is referred to as the Roux-en-Y gastric bypass (RYGB), the most commonly performed bariatric procedure in the United

States today (Fig. 9). The standard RYGB achieves weight loss primarily by restriction of food intake, which results from the creation of a small (15 to 30 cm³) gastric pouch with a 1-cm outlet. Malabsorption with the RYGB is due to bypass of the fundus, duodenum, and proximal jejunum, whereas nutrients bypass most of the bowel with the BPD procedure. It is important to recognize that there are more malabsorptive versions of the gastric bypass, the long-limb RYGB (Roux limb>150 cm) and the distal RYGB (common channel<100 cm), which typically are reserved for patients with BMIs exceeding 50 kg/m² [58].

Staged procedures

The highest-risk patients, including those with severe comorbidities and BMIs exceeding 60 kg/m², often are approached best in a staged fashion. At the initial stage, a sleeve gastrectomy is performed, which restricts food intake. Following a 200-lb or more weight loss, the patient returns to the operating room for conversion to a DS or RYGB procedure [59].

The minimally invasive approach

The first laparoscopic RYGB was reported in 1994 [60]. Using small incisions, the benefits of the laparoscopic approach include shorter hospitalization, decreased postoperative pain, earlier return to normal activity, reduced adhesion formation, and decreased incidence of incisional hernia, cardiopulmonary complications, and postoperative ileus [61]. Laparoscopy has become the most common method for performing bariatric surgery (Fig. 10). Compared with the open method, there is a slightly different profile for postoperative complications, including

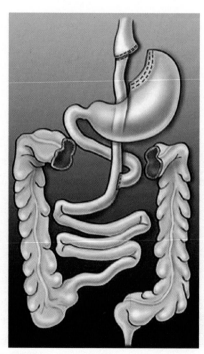

Fig. 9. The Roux-en-Y gastric bypass. (*Courtesy of* the American Society for Bariatric Surgery, Gainesville, FL; with permission.)

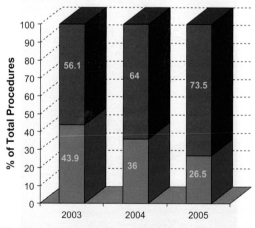

Fig. 10. Breakdown of laparoscopic versus open bariatric procedures in the United States. Blue shading, laparoscopic. Green shading, open. (*Data from* American Society for Bariatric Surgery, Gainesville, FL; with permission.)

a higher risk for anastomotic strictures and internal hernias leading to bowel obstruction [62].

Future directions

One of the most promising innovations is gastric pacing, in which electrodes stimulate the gastric antrum to produce satiety and weight loss [63]. There also have been trials with endoscopic placement of an intragastric balloon, which may have its greatest role in the high-risk superobese patient as a staged approach toward weight loss [64].

United States trends in bariatric surgery

The choice of procedure depends on several factors (**Box 2**), including surgeon and patient preference [65]. At present, the most common procedures performed in the United States are the laparoscopic RYGB and the Lap-Band procedure (**Fig. 11**). With a significant number of individuals classified as superobese, a consistent number of malabsorptive procedures are performed on an annual basis, including the long-limb gastric bypass and BPD/DS procedures (**Fig. 12**). These procedures place patients at the highest risk for long-term nutritional complications.

The postoperative course

It is helpful to have an understanding of the typical early and late postoperative course in evaluating the patient who has undergone bariatric surgery and sustained MWL. The first year following bariatric surgery is a critical period. Guidelines for follow-up care include an early postoperative visit during the first couple of weeks, and then at 3 months, 6 months, yearly for 3 years, and at 5-year intervals for life [66]. This follow-up varies as dictated by the patient's condition as well as requirements for band adjustments in patients with an adjustable gastric band.

A multidisciplinary approach is essential to the short and long-term care of the patient who has undergone bariatric surgery [67]. This involves collaboration and communication among the various health care professionals providing care, including

Box 2: Factors influencing choice of bariatric procedure
BMI
Age
Comorbid conditions
Eating habits
Cost
Patient preference
Surgeon preference

the bariatric surgeon, plastic surgeon, medical obesity specialist, registered dietician, and psychologist.

Early (up to 1 year)

During the first few months of rapid weight loss, defined as weight loss exceeding 1.5 kg or 1.5% of body weight per week [68], patients are at particular risk for developing dehydration, anemia, and gallstones. Nausea and vomiting often result from dysfunctional eating behavior, such as not chewing food completely or eating and drinking too fast. Patients essentially need to relearn how to eat. Without proper behavior modification, structural defects can develop, such as esophageal dilation with the band, dilatation of the gastric pouch, or slippage of the band. Nausea and vomiting also can result from a stricture or small bowel obstruction and may exacerbate dehydration.

Dumping syndrome

Often experienced by patients who have undergone gastric bypass, dumping syndrome refers to a group of unpleasant symptoms (nausea, palpitations, flushing, abdominal pain, diarrhea) related to the rapid emptying of stomach contents with high osmotic load into the small intestine [69]. This can be lessened by avoiding foods with a high sugar content and minimizing liquid intake with meals.

Anemia

Patients, especially menstruating women, frequently develop anemia [70]. Typically, this is an iron-deficiency anemia that results from a combination of blood loss from surgery, decreased iron intake, and, in the case of the gastric bypass, decreased absorption that is due to lack of gastric acidity in the newly created pouch. Any ongoing blood loss from the gastrointestinal tract, especially at the anastomotic site, needs to be ruled out. Patients often are provided supplemental liquid or chewable iron preparations.

Diet progression

The postbariatric surgery diet typically progresses over a 2-month period in a series of five to six stages, beginning with liquids and then with progressive increases in texture [71,72]. Adequate protein intake is important during the weight loss period to preserve lean body mass [73]. Requirements are calculated for the patient, with the adequacy of intake assessed by measuring serum albumin and changes in body composition with bioimpedance analysis.

Exercise

It is important for patients to begin an exercise program to preserve lean body mass. Initial exercise is

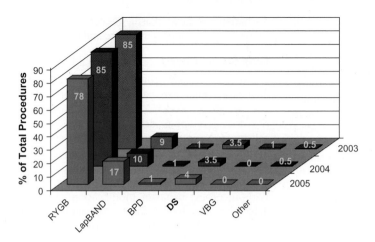

Fig. 11. Breakdown of bariatric procedures performed in the United States. (*Data from* American Society for Bariatric Surgery, Gainesville, FL; with permission.)

of mild intensity and performed on a regular basis, usually by walking and resistance training. Normally, 25% of weight lost by dieting alone is lean body mass; however, studies have shown that regular exercise can decrease this loss by up to 50% [74]. In the absence of physical activity, there is a risk for losing too much lean body mass, which can result in excessive hair loss, dry skin, easy bruising, brittle finger nails, reduced resistance to infection, increased risk for blood clots, less overall weight loss, and poor cardiovascular fitness.

Comorbidities

Most of the comorbidities will have improved significantly, if not resolved entirely, within the first 2 to 5 months following surgery [34]. Patients usually have a sleep study repeated to document resolution of sleep apnea. Obesity-related hypertension and type 2 diabetes also are likely to have resolved.

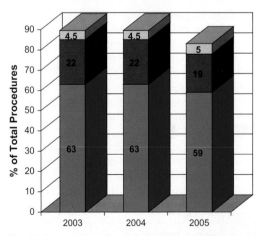

Fig. 12. Percentage of malabsorptive procedures performed in the United States. Lavender, DS/BPD diversion; blue, long-limb RYGB; green, RYGB. (*Data from* American Society for Bariatric Surgery, Gainesville, FL; with permission.)

Nausea and vomiting could still be a significant issue and should prompt further investigation with a swallow study or upper endoscopy to rule out stricture or small bowel obstruction. Inappropriate eating behavior often is an issue and requires ongoing dietary and psychologic support.

By the 6- to 12-month period, protein intake usually is no longer an issue, and patients usually are eating three meals per day consisting of a variety of foods. Weight loss may begin to plateau during this time, and activities that include more strength training and aerobic exercises are included. At this point, wound healing capacity, resistance to infection, and tolerance to stress is beginning to normalize.

Late (>1 year)

Even if all comorbid disease has resolved, patients should be reevaluated at a minimum on an annual basis. The long-term effects of some of these procedures are still not well defined; in particular, the Lap-Band experience in the United States is less than 10 years old. Malabsorptive procedures, such as the BPD, have long-term risk for loss of fat-soluble vitamins, osteomalacia, and protein malnutrition. The gastric bypass places patients at long-term risk for vitamin B_{12} and iron deficiency and osteoporosis. Additionally, continued monitoring for changes in lifestyle is vital to ensuring long-term success.

Weight loss results

Weight loss following bariatric surgery is reported often as percent excess weight loss (EWL). Excess weight is calculated as the difference between the patient's weight and the "ideal weight," taken from the 1983 Metropolitan Life Insurance Company data [75]. Success is defined often as 50% EWL [32,76]. The American Society for Bariatric Surgery also has recommended using postoperative BMI change as a parameter in evaluating bariatric surgery outcomes [77].

The RYGB is considered the gold standard with regard to weight loss results. Few patients reach normal weight, with most losing between 70% and 80% of their excess weight within the first 1 to 2 years [61,78,79]. Subsequently, there can be up to a 20% weight regain [31], with EWL at 5 years settling between 50% and 70% [80–82]. Results for patients who undergo BPD/DS are slightly better, with 75% EWL at 10 years [83]. With the lap BAND, early data suggest that maximum weight loss occurs only at 3 to 4 years, which takes considerably longer than with the gastric bypass or BPD. Long-term results are respectable, with 53% to 57% EWL at 5 to 6 years [84].

Evaluation and work-up

Many patients will present for body-contouring procedures as weight loss stabilizes between 12 and 18 months following bariatric surgery. A significant number will have been lost to follow-up by their bariatric surgeon [85], despite the need for long-term evaluation. Often, patients have been successful with weight loss and neglect to return for continued care [86]. Therefore, given the long-term physiologic and metabolic changes that challenge the patient who has undergone bariatric surgery and sustained MWL, a comprehensive preoperative evaluation is mandatory because these procedures often are extensive, with the potential for significant morbidity and even mortality [1,87,88]. There should be a low threshold for recommending treatment or referral to a specialist in preparing the patient who has undergone bariatric surgery and sustained MWL for body-contouring surgery.

Weight loss history

It is important to obtain an adequate history regarding the type of bariatric procedure, because the risk for various nutritional deficiencies can differ. This includes a history of any postoperative complications, such as thromboembolic disease, which could pose a risk for subsequent operations. Ideally, patients should be within 10% to 15% of their goal weight, with no more than a 1- to 2-lb per month fluctuation over a 3- to 6-month period. Patients who have settled well above their goal weight or those who have experienced significant weight regain should be referred back to their bariatric program. Often, they require additional dietary counseling or psychologic support, and, on occasion, may be candidates for revisional bariatric surgery. Lastly, patients with higher BMIs (>32 kg/m^2) tend to achieve suboptimal esthetic results [89,90]. There also is an increased risk for complications, especially as BMI exceeds 35 kg/m^2 [91].

Diet and exercise habits

An evaluation of the patient's diet and exercise habits also is important, including compliance with taking nutritional supplements. Persistent nausea or recurrent vomiting should prompt referral to the bariatric program for further evaluation for mechanical problems, including band slippage in Lap-Band patients. A review of the patient's exercise routine and capacity often is a good indicator of one's level of fitness for major surgery.

Residual medical problems

More often than not, the patient reports complete resolution of several comorbidities that were present before surgery. Nevertheless, it is important to inquire about residual problems or chronic disease states that could affect the safety of major body-contouring procedures. Bariatric consultants who know the patient well often are the best resource to aid in this evaluation.

Physical examination

Although the examination focuses on deformities of functional and esthetic concern, it is important to perform a complete physical examination. Particular attention should be directed toward identifying the location and reducibility of incisional hernias, as well as any signs of nutritional deficiency, including brittle nails, nystagmus, mucous membrane pallor, and atrophic glossitis. For Lap-Band patients, the access port should be palpated, with its location documented. The port often requires relocation on the abdominal wall during an abdominoplasty procedure. Ideally, this should be discussed and coordinated with the bariatric surgeon.

Laboratory work and studies

Laboratory work and preoperative studies should be obtained several weeks before surgery, which will guide the need for additional investigation and allow any abnormalities to be addressed in a timely fashion (Box 3).

Box 3:   Preoperative evaluation

Complete blood cell count
Electrolytes
Prothrombin/partial thromboplastin time
Albumin
Micronutrients[a]
12-Lead ECG[b]
Chest radiograph[b]

[a] Guided by history, physical examination, and type of bariatric procedure.
[b] Obtained when deemed necessary by surgeon or anesthesiologist

Late complications

The potential complications following bariatric surgery are numerous and are categorized as early and late. Major early complications include anastomotic leak and pulmonary embolism, both of which contribute to mortality [92]. More concerning to the plastic surgeon are the potential late complications, of which nutritional deficiencies predominate (Fig. 13) [93–95]. Patients who adhere to regular follow-up with their bariatric program are less likely to experience long-term complications.

There is significant variability in the literature regarding the incidence of various macro- and micronutrient deficiencies. They often only become evident years after surgery and frequently are underestimated and undertreated following bariatric surgery [96,97]. In some cases, patients may be chronically malnourished if they have not received regular evaluation or have been noncompliant with nutritional supplementation, which may occur as the weight comes off and patients begin to feel better.

Although procedures with a malabsorptive component place patients at greatest risk for malnutrition, it is important to recognize that all forms of bariatric surgery can lead to nutritional deficit [98]. Thus, patients with purely restrictive procedures may develop maladaptive eating behavior that can result in poor nutrient intake. In the setting of intractable vomiting, metabolic derangements can develop. Additionally, certain patients, particularly those with a history of binge-eating disorder, may make poor dietary choices by primarily consuming soft, high-calorie liquids foods (ice cream, milk shakes) that carry little nutritional value [99].

Macronutrient deficiency

Protein is the primary macronutrient at risk following bariatric surgery, with a reported incidence of deficiency up to 21% following malabsorptive procedures [100,101]. With rapid weight loss, the amino acid pool is diverted to gluconeogenesis, which, in combination with malabsorption and intolerance to high-protein foods, can lead to significant protein depletion [102]. A deficiency is evidenced by measurement of serum albumin, which, when observed with low serum phosphorus, indicates depletion of total body proteins. Albumin is a strong predictor of risk for adverse surgical outcome; a decrease in serum albumin from 46 g/L to less than 21 g/L is associated with increased morbidity and mortality, in particular due to sepsis and major infections [103]. In severe cases of deficiency with protein-energy malnutrition, hospitalization may be necessary for hyperalimentation, and refractory cases may require surgery to lengthen the common channel [50]. Response to protein supplementation is best assessed with serial prealbumin levels [104].

Dietary sources of high-quality protein should provide a minimum of 60 g, or 1 to 1.5 g/kg ideal body weight, daily [102]. Liquid protein

- Anastomotic Strictures
- Marginal Ulcers
- Nutritional Deficiency
- Incisional Hernia
- Internal Hernia
- Cholelithiasis
- Weight Regain
- Late Gastrointestinal Hemorrhage
- Liver Abnormalities
- Nephrolithiasis
- Band Erosion
- Mechanical Failure of Band

- Iron
    - Microcytic anemia, fatigue
- Vitamin B-12
    - Megaloblastic anemia, weakness, depression, peripheral neuropath
- Folate
    - Thrombocytopenia, glossitis
- Calcium
    - Inceased anesthetic risk, osteoporosis
- Vitamin A
    - Nightblindness, dry skin
- Vitamin D
    - Osteomalacia
- Zinc
    - Poor wound healing, hair loss
- Thiamin
    - Wernicke's polyneuropathy
- Protein
    - Poor wound healing, protein-calorie malnutrition

Fig. 13. Late complications.
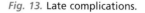

supplements may be necessary to fulfill this requirement. Wound healing from major surgery can increase protein requirements by up to 25% [105]. Therefore, even patients with a normal preoperative albumin level may be at risk postoperatively in the setting of malabsorption. Bioimpedance analysis is a tool used by many bariatric programs to measure body composition [106,107]. Ideally, women should have lean body mass greater than 75%, and men should have lean body mass greater than 80% [108]. Any concern regarding the adequacy of protein intake should prompt evaluation by a bariatric nutritionist.

Micronutrient deficiency

Iron Iron deficiency is observed following restrictive and malabsorptive procedures, with patients often having intolerance to red meat. The reported incidence in the literature is up to 47%, although figures vary depending on follow-up and the type of procedure [109]. Those at particular risk have a chronic source of blood loss, such as menstruation or stomal ulceration. Iron deficiency tends to worsen over time, with a peak incidence at 3 to 4 years. Iron studies should be evaluated in the setting of anemia, because iron deficiency anemia is common following gastric bypass. Iron deficiency usually is treated best with oral supplementation using ferrous sulfate, 200 mg three times a day [110], with the addition of vitamin C to enhance absorption [111].

Vitamin B_{12} Vitamin B_{12} is an important coenzyme in amino acid metabolism, and up to one third of patients with a gastric bypass will develop deficiency [109,112], setting the stage for macrocytic anemia and potentially irreversible neurologic sequelae. A low serum B_{12} level in combination with macrocytic red cells is indicative of a significant deficiency. Following gastric bypass, patients typically are supplemented with 500 to 600 µg daily. Deficient patients may require intramuscular injection of 1000 µg monthly, until liver stores are replenished.

Folate Folate is an essential water-soluble vitamin that acts as a coenzyme in the production of DNA, RNA, and amino acids. Deficiency occurs in up to 38% of patients following gastric bypass [113], leading to megaloblastic anemia and increased risk for neural tube defects during pregnancy. Folate deficiency is prevented easily with a minimum of 400 µg of daily dietary supplementation [109], typically the amount contained in a multivitamin.

Fasting serum levels of the amino acid homocysteine are elevated with weight loss [114]. This is a known risk factor for myocardial infarction, stroke, and thromboembolic disease [115].

Supplementation with adequate amounts of vitamin B_{12} and folate, essential cofactors in homocysteine metabolism, can normalize this level [114,116].

Thiamine (vitamin B_1) This water-soluble B vitamin is essential for amino acid and carbohydrate metabolism. Total body stores are approximately 30 mg, with a biologic half-life of about 15 days. Although routine multivitamin supplementation usually is adequate, patients can develop clinical symptoms of thiamine deficiency in less than 3 weeks with deficient intake. Significant deficiency usually is found in the setting of protracted nausea and vomiting. Early symptoms of deficiency include generalized weakness, ataxia, and numbness in the extremities. Thiamine deficiency leads to an elevation in the red blood cell transketolase, which is the best laboratory test for establishing a diagnosis [117]. Treatment is with 100 mg/d thiamine parenterally for 7 days. If untreated, thiamine deficiency can lead to Wernicke-Korsakoff's encephalopathy, which is characterized by mental confusion, memory loss, progressive paralysis, coma, and even death. Thiamine treatment should be instituted promptly, 100 mg intravenously, and continuing with 100 mg every 8 hours until there is resolution of symptoms [118]. In many cases, this occurs in as little as 24 hours, but it may take as long as 4 months. It is important to recognize that the administration of glucose and other carbohydrates without thiamine replacement can be dangerous in deficient states by precipitating central nervous system deterioration [119].

Calcium and vitamin D Calcium and vitamin D metabolism are linked tightly. Clinically significant deficiencies are seen most often following malabsorptive procedures [120]. Patients should receive 1200 to 1500 mg of calcium citrate and 800 IU vitamin D per day [121] to avoid deficiency, which can lead to metabolic bone disease [122] with an increased long-term risk for osteoporosis and fractures. Screening for deficiency includes evaluation of ionized calcium and vitamin D levels, alkaline phosphatase, and parathyroid hormone [123], as well as bone density studies.

Other fat-soluble vitamins Deficiencies in vitamins A, E, and K are seen most often following the BPD procedure, where there is malabsorption of fat [120]. There are reports of night blindness that is due to vitamin A deficiency; for this reason, some bariatric surgeons routinely supplement with higher doses of vitamin A. Vitamin E deficiency is not reported commonly. Vitamin K supplementation is recommended if the international normalized ratio exceeds 1.4 [124].

Other mineral and trace elements Zinc is not a commonly reported deficiency following bariatric procedures, although it also is not monitored routinely; a few published reports cite a prevalence as high as 50% following primarily malabsorptive procedures [120]. Deficiency has been linked with hair loss [125], although a greater concern is the potential effect on wound healing. Most patients do not receive zinc supplementation above the amount contained in a multivitamin.

Copper is an important cofactor for enzymes vital to functioning of the nervous system. Reported deficiency is rare, although it has been known to lead to demyelinating neuropathy and sideroblastic anemia [126–128]. Copper screening should be included for patients who present with neurologic deficits.

Electrolyte imbalances consisting primarily of hypokalemia and hypomagnesemia have been reported following gastric bypass [61,129].

Patient expectations and psychosocial issues

Considerable time is spent at the initial consultation with the patient who has sustained MWL and is a candidate for body-contouring surgery. It is important to evaluate expectations and motivations for seeking surgery. Although most will trade significant deformity and functional problems for lengthy and often visible scars, it is important to review the exact placement of these scars with the patient. Often, multiple body areas need to be addressed, and issues regarding staging and length of recovery should be discussed within the framework of the patient's social support network.

Most patients who have sustained MWL have enjoyed dramatic improvement in their medical condition and quality of life. Nevertheless, there is potential for significant postoperative psychiatric difficulty [91], and any untreated or poorly controlled psychiatric illness should prompt referral for further evaluation and treatment.

Summary

An understanding of the various bariatric surgical procedures is important in evaluating the patient for body-contouring procedures. The preoperative work-up of the patient who has sustained MWL should be comprehensive, with a focus on weight loss method and history and a search for any residual disease. Often, the multidisciplinary bariatric program can serve as an excellent referral source in the work-up of these patients. It is important to evaluate a patient's current lifestyle, including dietary protein sources and exercise tolerance. Late nutritional complications occur with significant

frequency and must be addressed in a timely fashion before surgery. Untreated or poorly controlled psychiatric illness should prompt referral for evaluation and treatment. Provided the necessary precautions are taken, the patient who has sustained MWL can be operated on safely. The benefit lies in being able to contribute to the patient's health and sense of well-being, with a high level of satisfaction that can be enjoyed by the patient and the surgeon.

References

[1] Shermak MA, Chang D, Magnuson TH, et al. An outcomes analysis of patients undergoing body contouring surgery after massive weight loss. Plast Reconstr Surg 2006;118(4):1026–31.

[2] Kamper MJ, Galloway DV, Ashley F. Abdominal panniculectomy after massive weight loss. Plast Reconstr Surg 1972;50(5):441–6.

[3] Zook EG. The massive weight loss patient. Clin Plast Surg 1975;2(3):457–66.

[4] McCraw LH Jr. Surgical rehabilitation after massive weight reduction. Case report. Plast Reconstr Surg 1974;53(3):349–52.

[5] Palmer B, Hallberg D, Backman L. Skin reduction plasties following intestinal shunt operations for treatment of obesity. Scand J Plast Reconstr Surg 1975;9(1):47–52.

[6] Centers for Disease Control and Prevention, Department of Health and Human Services. Overweight and obesity: obesity trends: U.S. Obesity Trends 1985–2005. Available at: http://www.cdc.gov/nccdphp/dnpa/obesity/trend/maps/index.htm. Accessed December 1, 2006.

[7] Inge TH, Garcia V, Daniels S, et al. A multidisciplinary approach to the adolescent bariatric surgical patient. J Pediatr Surg 2004;39(3):442–7 [discussion: 446–7].

[8] Hensrud DD, Klein S. Extreme obesity: a new medical crisis in the United States. Mayo Clin Proc 2006;81(10 Suppl):S5–10.

[9] National Institutes of Health, National Heart, Lung, and Blood Institute. Clinical guidelines on the identification, evaluation, and treatment of overweight and obesity in adults, the evidence report. Available at: http://www.nhlbi.nih.gov/guidelines/obesity/ob_gdlns.pdf. Accessed November 15, 2006.

[10] Renquist K. Obesity classification. Obes Surg 1997;7c(6):523.

[11] Stunkard AJ, Wadden TA. Obesity. Theory and therapy. 2nd edition. New York: Raven Press; 1993.

[12] Bray GA. Risks of obesity. Endocrinol Metab Clin North Am 2003;32(4):787–804, viii.

[13] Calle EE, Thun MJ, Petrelli JM, et al. Body-mass index and mortality in a prospective cohort of U.S. adults. N Engl J Med 1999;341(15):1097–105.

[14] U.S. Department of Health and Human Services. The Surgeon General's Call to Action to Prevent and Decrease Overweight and Obesity.

Rockville, MD: US Department of Health and Human Services, Public Health Service, Office of the Surgeon General; 2001.

[15] Lakka H, Bouchard C. Etiology of obesity. In: Buchwald H, Cowan GS Jr, Pories W, editors. Surgical management of obesity. Philadelphia: Saunders Elsevier; 2007. p. 18–28.

[16] Klein S. Medical management of obesity. Surg Clin North Am 2001;81(5):1025–38, v.

[17] National Institutes of Health, National Heart, Lung, and Blood Institute. NHLBI Education Initiative. The practical guide: identification, evaluation and treatment of overweight and obesity in adults. Available at: http://nhlbi.nih.gov/guidelines/obesity/prctgd_c.pdf. Accessed November 15, 2006.

[18] Wing RR, Blair E, Marcus M, et al. Year-long weight loss treatment for obese patients with type II diabetes: does including an intermittent very-low-calorie diet improve outcome? Am J Med 1994;97(4):354–62.

[19] Kennedy ET, Bowman SA, Spence JT, et al. Popular diets: correlation to health, nutrition, and obesity. J Am Diet Assoc 2001;101(4):411–20.

[20] Freedman MR, King J, Kennedy E. Popular diets: a scientific review. Obes Res 2001;9(Suppl 1): 1S–40S.

[21] Bravata DM, Sanders L, Huang J, et al. Efficacy and safety of low-carbohydrate diets: a systematic review. JAMA 2003;289(14):1837–50.

[22] Cowan GS Jr. Nonsurgical methods of weight loss. In: Buchwald H, Cowan GS Jr, Pories W, editors. Surgical management of obesity. Philadelphia: Saunders Elsevier; 2007. p. 83–90.

[23] Garrow JS, Summerbell CD. Meta-analysis: effect of exercise, with or without dieting, on the body composition of overweight subjects. Eur J Clin Nutr 1995;49(1):1–10.

[24] Wing RR, Hill JO. Successful weight loss maintenance. Annu Rev Nutr 2001;21:323–41.

[25] Connolly HM, Crary JL, McGoon MD, et al. Valvular heart disease associated with fenfluramine-phentermine. N Engl J Med 1997;337 (9):581–8.

[26] Padwal RS, Majumdar SR. Drug treatments for obesity: orlistat, sibutramine, and rimonabant. Lancet 2007;369(9555):71–7.

[27] Drenick EJ, Johnson D. Weight reduction by fasting and semistarvation in morbid obesity: long-term follow-up. Int J Obes 1978;2(2): 123–32.

[28] Anderson JW, Konz EC, Frederich RC, et al. Long-term weight-loss maintenance: a meta-analysis of US studies. Am J Clin Nutr 2001; 74(5):579–84.

[29] Brolin RE. Update: NIH Consensus Conference. Gastrointestinal surgery for severe obesity. Nutrition 1996;12(6):403–4.

[30] Buchwald H, Buchwald JN. Evolution of operative procedures for the management of morbid obesity 1950–2000. Obes Surg 2002;12(5): 705–17.

[31] Pories WJ, Swanson MS, MacDonald KG, et al. Who would have thought it? An operation proves to be the most effective therapy for adult-onset diabetes mellitus. Ann Surg 1995; 222(3):339–50 [discussion: 350–2].

[32] Christou NV, Sampalis JS, Liberman M, et al. Surgery decreases long-term mortality, morbidity, and health care use in morbidly obese patients. Ann Surg 2004;240(3):416–23 [discussion 423–4].

[33] National Institutes of Health Consensus Development Panel. National Institutes of Health consensus development conference statement, gastrointestinal conference statement, gastrointestinal surgery for severe obesity. Ann Intern Med 1991;115:956–61.

[34] Buchwald H. Consensus conference statement bariatric surgery for morbid obesity: health implications for patients, health professionals, and third-party payers. Surg Obes Relat Dis 2005;1(3):371–81.

[35] Kremen AJ, Linner JH, Nelson CH. An experimental evaluation of the nutritional importance of proximal and distal small intestine. Ann Surg 1954;140(3):439–48.

[36] Payne JH, Dewind LT, Commons RR. Metabolic observations in patients with jejunocolic shunts. Am J Surg 1963;106:273–89.

[37] Lewis LA, Turnbull RB Jr, Page IH. Effects of jejunocolic shunt on obesity, serum lipoproteins, lipids, and electrolytes. Arch Intern Med 1966;117(1):4–16.

[38] Lewis LA, Turnbull RB Jr, Page IH. "Short-circuiting" of the small intestine. Effect on concentration of serum cholesterol and lipoproteins. JAMA 1962;182:77–9.

[39] Scott HW Jr, Sandstead HH, Brill AB, et al. Experience with a new technique of intestinal bypass in the treatment of morbid obesity. Ann Surg 1971;174(4):560–72.

[40] Payne JH, DeWind LT. Surgical treatment of obesity. Am J Surg 1969;118(2):141–7.

[41] Buchwald H, Rucker RD. The rise and fall of jejunoileal bypass. In: Nelson R, Nyhus LM, editors. Surgery of the small intestine. Norwalk (CT): Appleton Century Crofts; 1987. p. 529–41.

[42] Deitel M. Jejunocolic and jejunoileal bypass: an historical perspective. In: Deitel M, editor. Surgery for the morbidly obese patient. Philadelphia: Lea and Febiger; 1998. p. 81–9.

[43] Printen KJ, Mason EE. Gastric surgery for relief of morbid obesity. Arch Surg 1973;106(4): 428–31.

[44] Pace WG, Martin EW Jr, Tetirick T, et al. Gastric partitioning for morbid obesity. Ann Surg 1979; 190(3):392–400.

[45] Laws HL, Piantadosi S. Superior gastric reduction procedure for morbid obesity: a prospective, randomized trial. Ann Surg 1981;193(3): 334–40.

[46] Eckhout GV, Willbanks OL, Moore JT. Vertical ring gastroplasty for morbid obesity. Five year

experience with 1,463 patients. Am J Surg 1986; 152(6):713–6.

[47] Mason EE. Vertical banded gastroplasty for obesity. Arch Surg 1982;117(5):701–6.

[48] Kuzmak LI. A review of seven years' experience with silicone gastric banding. Obes Surg 1991; 1(4):403–8.

[49] Scopinaro N, Gianetta E, Pandolfo N, et al. [Bilio-pancreatic bypass. Proposal and preliminary experimental study of a new type of operation for the functional surgical treatment of obesity]. Minerva Chir 1976;31(10):560–6.

[50] Hess DS, Hess DW. Biliopancreatic diversion with a duodenal switch. Obes Surg 1998;8(3): 267–82.

[51] Scopinaro N, Gianetta E, Civalleri D, et al. Two years of clinical experience with biliopancreatic bypass for obesity. Am J Clin Nutr 1980;33 (2 Suppl):506–14.

[52] Mason EE. Historical perspectives. In: Buchwald H, Cowan GS Jr, Pories W, editors. Surgical management of obesity. Philadelphia: Saunders Elsevier; 2007. p. 3–9.

[53] Mason EE, Ito C. Gastric bypass in obesity. Surg Clin North Am 1967;47(6):1345–51.

[54] Torres JC, Oca CF, Garrison RN. Gastric bypass: Roux-en-Y gastrojejunostomy from the lesser curvature. South Med J 1983;76(10):1217–21.

[55] Fobi M. Why the operation I prefer is silastic ring vertical gastric bypass. Obes Surg 1991; 1(4):423–6.

[56] Brolin RE, Kenler HA, Gorman JH, et al. Long-limb gastric bypass in the superobese. A prospective randomized study. Ann Surg 1992; 215(4):387–95.

[57] Griffen WO Jr, Young VL, Stevenson CC. A prospective comparison of gastric and jejunoileal bypass procedures for morbid obesity. Ann Surg 1977;186(4):500–9.

[58] MacLean LD, Rhode BM, Nohr CW. Late outcome of isolated gastric bypass. Ann Surg 2000;231(4):524–8.

[59] Regan JP, Inabnet WB, Gagner M, et al. Early experience with two-stage laparoscopic Roux-en-Y gastric bypass as an alternative in the super-super obese patient. Obes Surg 2003;13(6): 861–4.

[60] Wittgrove AC, Clark GW, Tremblay LJ. Laparoscopic gastric bypass, Roux-en-Y: preliminary report of five cases. Obes Surg 1994;4(4): 353–7.

[61] Schauer PR, Ikramuddin S, Gourash W, et al. Outcomes after laparoscopic Roux-en-Y gastric bypass for morbid obesity. Ann Surg 2000; 232(4):515–29.

[62] Rogula T, Brethauer SA, Thodiyil PA, et al. Current status of laparoscopic gastric bypass. In: Buchwald H, Cowan GS Jr, Pories W, editors. Surgical management of obesity. Philadelphia: Saunders Elsevier; 2007. p. 191–203.

[63] Cigaina VV, Pinato G, Rigo VV, et al. Gastric peristalsis control by mono situ electrical

stimulation: a preliminary study. Obes Surg 1996;6(3):247–9.

[64] Spyropoulos C, Katsakoulis E, Mead N, et al. Intragastric balloon for high-risk super-obese patients: a prospective analysis of efficacy. Surg Obes Relat Dis 2007;3(1):78–83.

[65] Salameh JR. Bariatric surgery: past and present. Am J Med Sci 2006;331(4):194–200.

[66] Mason EE, Amaral JF, Cowan GS Jr, et al. Guidelines for selection of patients for surgical treatment of obesity. Obes Surg 1993;3(4):429.

[67] McMahon MM, Sarr MG, Clark MM, et al. Clinical management after bariatric surgery: value of a multidisciplinary approach. Mayo Clin Proc 2006;81(10 Suppl):S34–45.

[68] Wadden T, Osei S. The treatment of obesity: an overview. In: Wadden T, Stunkard AJ, editors. Handbook of obesity treatment. New York: Guilford Press; 2002. p. 229–49.

[69] Pories WJ, Caro JF, Flickinger EG, et al. The control of diabetes mellitus (NIDDM) in the morbidly obese with the Greenville gastric bypass. Ann Surg 1987;206(3):316–23.

[70] Brolin RE, Gorman JH, Gorman RC, et al. Prophylactic iron supplementation after Roux-en-Y gastric bypass: a prospective, double-blind, randomized study. Arch Surg 1998;133(7): 740–4.

[71] Saltzman E, Anderson W, Apovian CM, et al. Criteria for patient selection and multidisciplinary evaluation and treatment of the weight loss surgery patient. Obes Res 2005;13(2):234–43.

[72] Marcason W. What are the dietary guidelines following bariatric surgery? J Am Diet Assoc 2004;104(3):487–8.

[73] Vazquez JA, Kazi U, Madani N. Protein metabolism during weight reduction with very-low-energy diets: evaluation of the independent effects of protein and carbohydrate on protein sparing. Am J Clin Nutr 1995;62(1):93–103.

[74] Ballor DL, Poehlman ET. Exercise-training enhances fat-free mass preservation during diet-induced weight loss: a meta-analytical finding. Int J Obes Relat Metab Disord 1994;18(1): 35–40.

[75] Deitel M, Greenstein RJ. Recommendations for reporting weight loss. Obes Surg 2003;13(2): 159–60.

[76] Halverson JD, Zuckerman GR, Koehler RE, et al. Gastric bypass for morbid obesity: a medical-surgical assessment. Ann Surg 1981;194(2): 152–60.

[77] Standards Committee, American Society for Bariatric Surgery. Guidelines for reporting results in bariatric surgery. Obes Surg 1997;7:521–2.

[78] DeMaria EJ, Sugerman HJ, Kellum JM, et al. Results of 281 consecutive total laparoscopic Roux-en-Y gastric bypasses to treat morbid obesity. Ann Surg 2002;235(5):640–5 [discussion: 645–7].

[79] Wittgrove AC, Clark GW. Laparoscopic gastric bypass, Roux-en-Y- 500 patients: technique

and results, with 3-60 month follow-up. Obes Surg 2000;10(3):233–9.

[80] Reinhold RB. Late results of gastric bypass surgery for morbid obesity. J Am Coll Nutr 1994; 13(4):326–31.

[81] Sugerman HJ, Kellum JM, Engle KM, et al. Gastric bypass for treating severe obesity. Am J Clin Nutr 1992;55(2 Suppl):560S–6S.

[82] White S, Brooks E, Jurikova L, et al. Long-term outcomes after gastric bypass. Obes Surg 2005;15(2):155–63.

[83] Hess DS, Hess DW, Oakley RS. The biliopancreatic diversion with the duodenal switch: results beyond 10 years. Obes Surg 2005;15(3): 408–16.

[84] Fielding GA, Ren CJ. Laparoscopic adjustable gastric band. Surg Clin North Am 2005;85(1): 129–40, x.

[85] Renquist K, Jeng G, Mason EE. Calculating follow-up rates. Obes Surg 1992;2(4):361–7.

[86] Oria HE. Reporting results in obesity surgery: evaluation of a limited survey. Obes Surg 1996;6(4):361–8.

[87] Rohrich RJ. Mastering shape and form in cosmetic surgery: the Annual Meeting of the American Society for Aesthetic Plastic Surgery. Plast Reconstr Surg 2001;108(3):741–2.

[88] Taylor J, Shermak M. Body contouring following massive weight loss. Obes Surg 2004; 14(8):1080–5.

[89] Nemerofsky RB, Oliak DA, Capella JF. Body lift: an account of 200 consecutive cases in the massive weight loss patient. Plast Reconstr Surg 2006;117(2):414–30.

[90] Aly AS, Cram AE, Chao M, et al. Belt lipectomy for circumferential truncal excess: the University of Iowa experience. Plast Reconstr Surg 2003;111(1):398–413.

[91] Aly AS, Cram AE, Heddens C. Truncal body contouring surgery in the massive weight loss patient. Clin Plast Surg 2004;31(4): 611–24, vii.

[92] Thodiyil PA, Rogula T, Mattar SG, et al. Management of complications after laparoscopic gastric bypass. In: Inabnet WB, DeMaria EJ, Ikramuddin S, editors. Laparoscopic bariatric surgery. Philadelphia: Lippincott Williams & Wilkins; 2005. p. 225–37.

[93] Bloomberg RD, Fleishman A, Nalle JE, et al. Nutritional deficiencies following bariatric surgery: what have we learned? Obes Surg 2005; 15(2):145–54.

[94] Ward DJ, Wilson JS. Abdominal reduction following jejunoileal bypass for morbid obesity. Br J Plast Surg 1989;42(5):586–90.

[95] Sanger C, David LR. Impact of significant weight loss on outcome of body-contouring surgery. Ann Plast Surg 2006;56(1):9–13 [discussion: 13].

[96] Skroubis G, Sakellaropoulos G, Pouggouras K, et al. Comparison of nutritional deficiencies after Roux-en-Y gastric bypass and after biliopancreatic diversion with Roux-en-Y gastric bypass. Obes Surg 2002;12(4):551–8.

[97] Brolin RE, Leung M. Survey of vitamin and mineral supplementation after gastric bypass and biliopancreatic diversion for morbid obesity. Obes Surg 1999;9(2):150–4.

[98] Byrne TK. Complications of surgery for obesity. Surg Clin North Am 2001;81(5):1181–93, vii–viii.

[99] Kalarchian MA, Marcus MD, Wilson GT, et al. Binge eating among gastric bypass patients at long-term follow-up. Obes Surg 2002;12(2): 270–5.

[100] Brolin RE, LaMarca LB, Kenler HA, et al. Malabsorptive gastric bypass in patients with superobesity. J Gastrointest Surg 2002;6(2):195–203 [discussion: 204–5].

[101] Scopinaro N, Gianetta E, Adami GF, et al. Biliopancreatic diversion for obesity at eighteen years. Surgery 1996;119(3):261–8.

[102] Moize V, Geliebter A, Gluck ME, et al. Obese patients have inadequate protein intake related to protein intolerance up to 1 year following Roux-en-Y gastric bypass. Obes Surg 2003; 13(1):23–8.

[103] Gibbs J, Cull W, Henderson W, et al. Preoperative serum albumin level as a predictor of operative mortality and morbidity: results from the National VA Surgical Risk Study. Arch Surg 1999;134(1):36–42.

[104] Beck FK, Rosenthal TC. Prealbumin: a marker for nutritional evaluation. Am Fam Physician 2002;65(8):1575–8.

[105] Van Way CW 3rd. Nutritional support in the injured patient. Surg Clin North Am 1991;71(3): 537–48.

[106] Livingston EH, Sebastian JL, Huerta S, et al. Biexponential model for predicting weight loss after gastric surgery for obesity. J Surg Res 2001;101(2):216–24.

[107] Madan AK, Kuykendall ST, Orth WS, et al. Does laparoscopic gastric bypass result in a healthier body composition? An affirmative answer. Obes Surg 2006;16(4):465–8.

[108] Raum WJ. Postoperative medical management of bariatric patients. In: Martin LF, editor. Obesity surgery. New York: McGraw-Hill; 2004. p. 133–59.

[109] Brolin RE, Gorman JH, Gorman RC, et al. Are vitamin B12 and folate deficiency clinically important after roux-en-Y gastric bypass? J Gastrointest Surg 1998;2(5):436–42.

[110] Goddard AF, McIntyre AS, Scott BB. Guidelines for the management of iron deficiency anaemia. British Society of Gastroenterology. Gut 2000; 46(Suppl 3–4):IV1–5.

[111] Rhode BM, Shustik C, Christou NV, et al. Iron absorption and therapy after gastric bypass. Obes Surg 1999;9(1):17–21.

[112] Yale CE, Gohdes PN, Schilling RF. Cobalamin absorption and hematologic status after two types of gastric surgery for obesity. Am J Hematol 1993;42(1):63–6.

[113] Mallory GN, Macgregor AM. Folate status following gastric bypass surgery (the great folate mystery). Obes Surg 1991;1(1):69–72.

[114] Dixon JB, Dixon ME, O'Brien PE. Elevated homocysteine levels with weight loss after Lap-Band surgery: higher folate and vitamin B12 levels required to maintain homocysteine level. Int J Obes Relat Metab Disord 2001; 25(2):219–27.

[115] Welch GN, Loscalzo J. Homocysteine and atherothrombosis. N Engl J Med 1998;338(15): 1042–50.

[116] Dixon JB. Elevated homocysteine with weight loss. Obes Surg 2001;11(5):537–8.

[117] Warnock LG. Transketolase activity of blood hemolysate, a useful index for diagnosing thiamine deficiency. Clin Chem 1975;21(3):432–6.

[118] Mason ME, Jalagani H, Vinik AI. Metabolic complications of bariatric surgery: diagnosis and management issues. Gastroenterol Clin North Am 2005;34(1):25–33.

[119] Sola E, Morillas C, Garzon S, et al. Rapid onset of Wernicke's encephalopathy following gastric restrictive surgery. Obes Surg 2003;13(4):661–2.

[120] Slater GH, Ren CJ, Siegel N, et al. Serum fat-soluble vitamin deficiency and abnormal calcium metabolism after malabsorptive bariatric surgery. J Gastrointest Surg 2004;8(1):48–55 [discussion: 54–5].

[121] Kushner R. Managing the obese patient after bariatric surgery: a case report of severe malnutrition and review of the literature. JPEN J Parenter Enteral Nutr 2000;24(2): 126–32.

[122] Parfitt AM, Miller MJ, Frame B, et al. Metabolic bone disease after intestinal bypass for treatment of obesity. Ann Intern Med 1978;89(2): 193–9.

[123] Goldner WS, O'Dorisio TM, Dillon JS, et al. Severe metabolic bone disease as a long-term complication of obesity surgery. Obes Surg 2002;12(5):685–92.

[124] Marceau P, Hould FS, Lebel S, et al. Malabsorptive obesity surgery. Surg Clin North Am 2001; 81(5):1113–27.

[125] Neve HJ, Bhatti WA, Soulsby C, et al. Reversal of hair loss following vertical gastroplasty when treated with zinc sulphate. Obes Surg 1996;6(1):63–5.

[126] Schleper B, Stuerenburg HJ. Copper deficiency-associated myelopathy in a 46-year-old woman. J Neurol 2001;248(8):705–6.

[127] Kumar N, McEvoy KM, Ahlskog JE. Myelopathy due to copper deficiency following gastrointestinal surgery. Arch Neurol 2003;60(12): 1782–5.

[128] Almhanna K, Khan P, Schaldenbrand M, et al. Sideroblastic anemia after bariatric surgery. Am J Hematol 2006;81(2):155–6.

[129] Halverson JD. Micronutrient deficiencies after gastric bypass for morbid obesity. Am Surg 1986;52(11):594–8.

CLINICS IN
PLASTIC
SURGERY

Clin Plastic Surg 35 (2008) 27–51

ELSEVIER
SAUNDERS

Body Lift

Joseph F. Capella, MD[a,b]

The abdomen, thighs, and buttocks are often the areas of greatest concern to patients following massive weight loss. The typical appearance of the patient who has lost a massive amount of weight derives from a combination of factors, including a gender-dependent body morphology and a change in body mass index (BMI), which lead to skin and soft tissue excess and poor skin tone. Women tend to have excess skin along the anterior abdominal wall, flank, and hip regions as well as cellulite and excess skin along the thighs and buttocks. The buttocks and pubic areas often are ptotic and redundant (Fig. 1) [1]. Men have similar changes to the abdominal, flank, hip, medial thigh, and pubic regions; however, the anterior, posterior, and lateral thighs and buttocks are affected to a lesser degree and usually are without cellulite (Fig. 2). The body contour stigmata of massive weight loss for men and women is the consequence of the skin and soft tissues failing to retract completely following the metabolism of fat through bariatric surgery or following lifestyle changes. The excess skin and soft tissues descend inferomedially from the characteristic areas of fat deposition. The fat deposits of the axilla and flank produce rolls along the upper and midback and flank. The hip fat deposit produces a roll just below the top of the iliac crest in men and often onto the proximal lateral thigh in women. The collapse of redundant tissues from the lower abdomen, mons pubis, and buttocks as well as the redundant tissues from the fat deposits of the medial thigh itself contribute directly to the excess tissues along the medial thighs. The descent of redundant tissues from the fat deposits circumferentially along the thighs in women creates the potential for skin folds throughout the thighs, resulting in both a vertical and horizontal tissue excess. Along with issues of skin and soft tissue excess, the patient who has undergone bariatric surgery tends to have deficiencies in skin tone. Obese individuals usually have been overweight since childhood and nearly always since adolescence [2]. The average age for bariatric procedures is 37 years [3]. In the years before gastric reduction procedures, obese individuals have typically gained and lost weight numerous times in attempts to lose weight through dieting or behavioral modification. The prolonged period of skin under

[a] Department of Plastic Surgery, Hackensack University Medical Center, Hackensack, NJ, USA
[b] Department of Surgery, University of Medicine and Dentistry of New Jersey, Newark, NJ, USA
E-mail address: jfcapella@aol.com

doi:10.1016/j.cps.2007.08.001

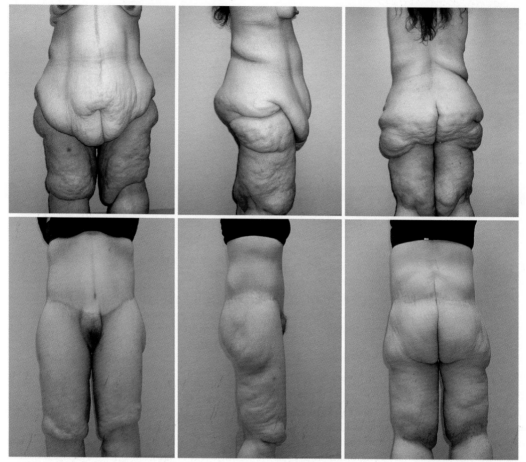

Fig. 1. (*Top*) Type III 40-year-old woman 40 months following tubular, banded gastric bypass surgery and weight loss of 269 lbs (122 kg). Current weight and BMI: 254 lbs (115 kg) and 41 kg/m², respectively. Maximum weight and BMI: 522 lbs (237 kg) and 84 kg/m², respectively. (*Bottom*) Twenty-five months following an abdominoplasty and circumferential thigh liposuction, 9 months following lower body lift, and 4 months following medial thigh lift with a vertical component.

tension and the frequent history of "yo-yo" dieting lead to poor skin elasticity following massive weight loss [4]. Striae and cellulite are common throughout the torso, particularly in women. The extreme body contour deformities that distinguish the routine patient from the patent who has lost a massive amount of weight has led to the development of operative techniques specific to these individuals.

The ideal body contouring procedure for the patient who has lost a massive amount of weight should effectively address all or as much of the characteristic stigmata in a safe, efficient, and consistent manner. Various techniques have been described to treat the postbariatric body condition; these include body lift, belt lipectomy, lower body lift, and circumferential torsoplasty [4–7]. Although they have different names, each involves a simultaneous abdominoplasty and thigh and

buttock lift. The goal of all of these procedures is to reverse or derotate the inferomedial collapse of the skin and soft tissues of the body (see Fig. 2). Aside from the obvious advantage of addressing the thighs and buttocks as well as the abdomen in one stage, a simultaneous circumferential procedure offers another important advantage: a standing cone is less of a concern. In excisional body contouring procedures, some graduation in the amount of skin to be excised must exist to prevent the formation of a standing cone or "dog ear" at the lateral extent of the scar (Fig. 3). Circumferential procedures allow for the appropriate amount of tissue to be excised from the areas being addressed. The surge in bariatric procedures in the United States and abroad over the last 5 years has led to increasing patient requests for body-contouring procedures [8]. To treat the postbariatric condition, some plastic surgeons are implementing

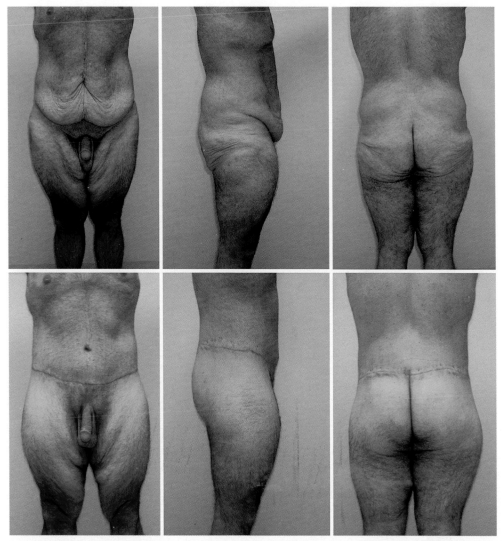

Fig. 2. (*Top*) Type III 30-year-old man 22 months following tubular, banded gastric bypass surgery and weight loss of 189 lbs (86 kg). Current weight and BMI: 213 lbs (97 kg) and 32 kg/m², respectively. Maximum weight and BMI: 403 lbs (183 kg) and 60 kg/m², respectively. (*Bottom*) Four months following body lift. The patient is a candidate for a medial thigh lift.

traditional procedures and others are performing more extensive circumferential approaches [4–7, 9–13]. Attempts to manage the patient who has undergone bariatric surgery with abdominoplasty and liposuction alone are likely to result in an unsatisfactory outcome (see Fig. 3; Figs. 4 and 5). Likewise, extending an abdominoplasty to be circumferential without thigh and buttock undermining usually produces less than optimal results. Many plastic surgeons have been reluctant to apply skin-tightening procedures to deformities of the thigh and buttock region because of poor scars, unreliable scar location, high complication rates, and the magnitude of these procedures [14]. Largely because of Lockwood's many important contributions

to body contouring and the increase in demand for these procedures, plastic surgeons are approaching postbariatric body contouring with renewed enthusiasm and interest [6,15–18]. By developing the lower body lift version I and later version II, Lockwood approached the abdomen, thighs, and buttocks as a unit, realizing that each of these areas of the body had to be treated effectively to produce the best overall outcome. Treating the abdomen, thighs, and buttocks as singular units would negate the powerful benefits of a circumferential procedure. Lockwood also emphasized the importance of approximating the superficial fascial system with permanent sutures to maintain soft tissue contour over the long-term and to maximize scar

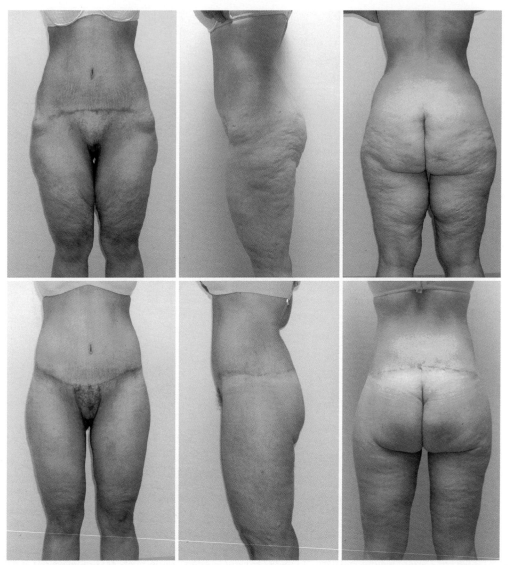

Fig. 3. (*Top*) Type I 34-year-old woman 19 months following abdominoplasty and prior weight loss of 166 lbs (75 kg) through lifestyle changes. Current weight and BMI: 167 lbs (76 kg) and 25 kg/m², respectively. Maximum weight and BMI: 345 lbs (157 kg) and 51 kg/m², respectively. (*Bottom*) Six months following lower body lift and 3 months following medial thigh lift with a vertical component.

quality. Our technique for addressing the abdomen, thighs, and buttocks in the patient who has lost a massive amount of weight is based on Lockwood's description of the lower body lift, version II; however, it differs in several ways, particularly with regard to our method of marking, choice for scar location, intraoperative patient positioning, and, recently, choice of suture material. In addition, we have chosen to call our technique a "body lift" rather than a "lower body lift." We prefer this term because it allows us to describe the procedures potentially available to our patients more accurately. For example, a "lower body lift" in our

practice is a circumferential thigh and buttock lift; it is similar to Lockwood's description of a lower body lift, version I, but without the medial thigh lift. We apply this technique commonly to patients who have lost weight and who already have undergone an abdominoplasty (see Figs. 3 and 5). We also believe that the term "body lift" describes our procedure better in that along with the lower body, the flank, back, and chest areas usually are affected to a large degree (Figs. 6 and 7). Our preference is to perform a body lift or simultaneous abdominoplasty and thigh and buttock lift on patients following massive weight loss when the

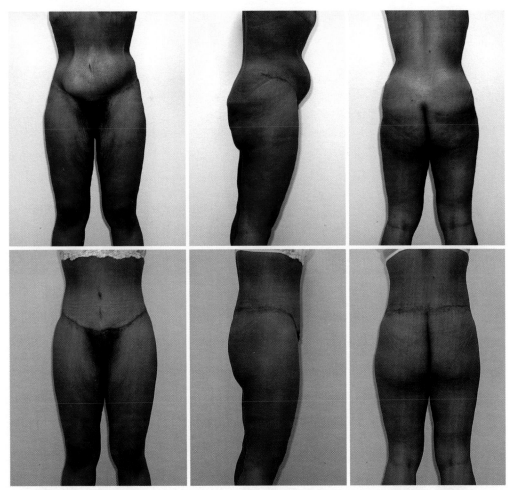

Fig. 4. (*Top*) Type I 34-year-old woman 21 months following tubular, banded gastric bypass surgery and panniculectomy and weight loss of 101 lbs (46 kg). Current weight and BMI: 143 lbs (65 kg) and 27 kg/m^2, respectively. Maximum weight and BMI: 242 lbs (110 kg) and 46 kg/m^2, respectively. (*Bottom*) Three months following body lift.

appropriate indications are present and when patient selection criteria have been met.

Patient selection

Proper patient selection is critical for maximizing the likelihood of a good outcome and minimizing complications following a body lift. Patients should be at a stable weight for several months and ideally at their lowest weight before surgery (Box 1). Following gastric bypass surgery, this may range from 1 to 2 years, depending on prebariatric weight. For example, following gastric bypass, a 200-kg man will take longer to stabilize in weight than will a 100-kg woman. Weight loss following gastric bypass surgery and other restrictive and malabsorptive procedures, such as biliopancreatic bypass, tends to be rapid during the first 8 to 12 postoperative months [3,19]. Weight loss following purely restrictive bariatric procedures, such as vertical-banded gastroplasty and gastric banding, tends to be less and slower, with weight loss achieved over periods of as long as 3 years [20,21]. The disadvantage of performing body-contouring procedures on patients with ongoing weight loss is the potential for early recurrence of tissue laxity. We avoid performing body lifts on individuals with a BMI of greater than 35 kg/m^2. Traction from the waistline in this population often has only a minimal effect on skin excess and cellulite along the lower buttocks and distal thighs. This heavier group of patients who have undergone bariatric surgeries typically has a large pannus present along the lower abdomen extending to the hips and tapering over the buttocks. Difficulty with activities, severe intertriginous dermatitis, and back discomfort usually

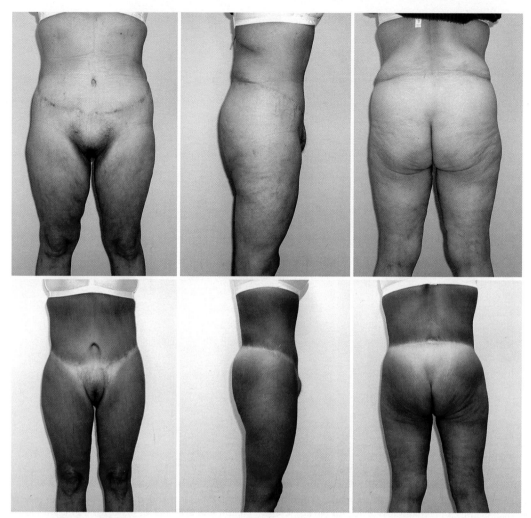

Fig. 5. (*Top*) Type I 59-year-old woman 46 months following tubular, banded gastric bypass surgery and weight loss of 86 lbs (39 kg) and 28 months following abdominoplasty. Current weight and BMI: 144 lbs (65 kg) and 26 kg/m², respectively. Maximum weight and BMI: 230 lbs (105 kg) and 42 kg/m², respectively. (*Bottom*) Twenty-six months following lower body lift and 3 months following medial thigh lift with a vertical component.

are their biggest complaints. We offer these patients a near circumferential abdominoplasty, a far less complex procedure. On occasion, we offer body lifts to this heavier group, particularly patients who are younger than 35 years of age, usually men, but also women who have a more central fat distribution. We avoid performing a body lift on a patient who has undergone bariatric surgery who is older than 55 years of age. Morbidly obese individuals who have sought bariatric surgery in the fifth and sixth decades of life often have developed degenerative arthritis and in many instances have undergone joint replacement. We find the recovery from body lifts in patients who have ongoing arthritis and following joint replacement to be

difficult and protracted. We usually offer this group an abdominoplasty or an abdominoplasty to be followed in 6 months by a thigh and buttock lift. Patients who have undergone bariatric surgery, particularly menstruating women and those who have had malabsorptive procedures (ie, gastric bypass and biliopancreatic bypass), often are anemic [22]. These anemias tend to be secondary to the poor absorption of iron and folate. Patients considering a body lift are encouraged to take an iron supplement and daily multivitamins. Severely anemic patients are referred to a hematologist. We prefer a baseline hemoglobin of 12. All patients who have undergone bariatric surgery are encouraged to continue follow-up with their bariatric surgeon.

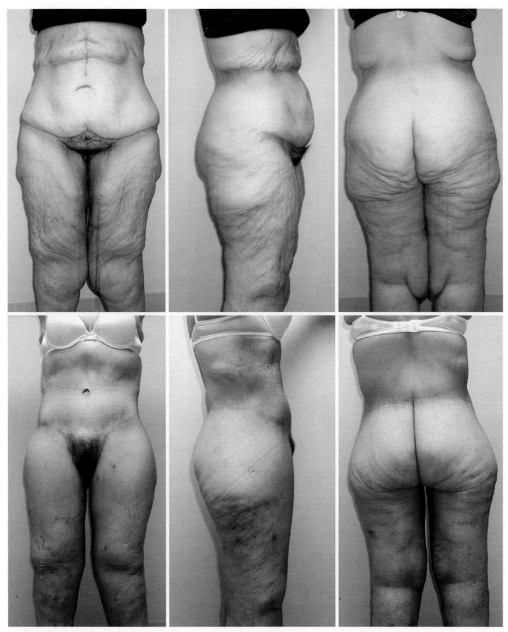

Fig. 6. (*Top*) Type II 55-year-old woman 13 months following tubular, banded gastric bypass surgery and weight loss of 115 lbs (52 kg). Current weight and BMI: 156 lbs (71 kg) and 30 kg/m², respectively. Maximum weight and BMI: 271 lbs (123 kg) and 53 kg/m², respectively. (*Bottom*) Twenty-two months following body lift and 10 months following medial thigh lift with a vertical component.

Surgical technique

The challenge of performing a consistently effective circumferential body–contouring procedure in the population who has lost a massive amount of weight relates directly to the properties inherent in this patient population and the objectives to be achieved. Skin and soft tissue excess and a high degree of skin and soft tissue mobility are common to all individuals who have lost a large amount of weight. Attempting to affect change to the upper abdomen or distal thighs from the level of the lower torso, the usual location for circumferential procedures, requires a significant degree of traction. The combination of these patient properties with high levels of traction leads to the potential for

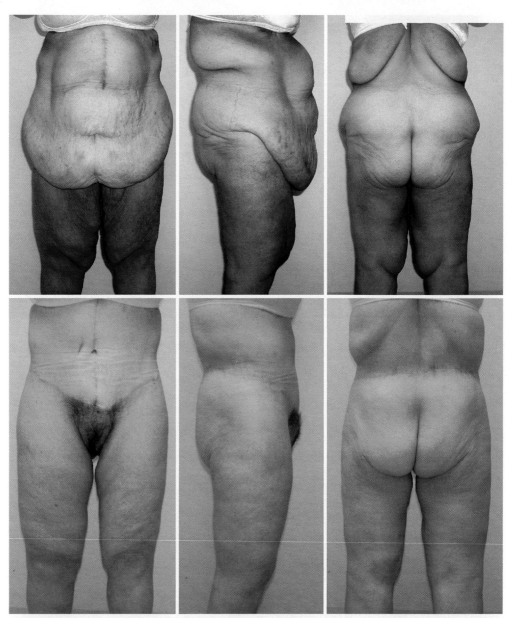

Fig. 7. (Top) Type III 55-year-old woman 13 months following tubular, banded gastric bypass surgery and weight loss of 154 lbs (70 kg). Current weight and BMI: 209 lbs (95 kg) and 35 kg/m², respectively. Maximum weight and BMI: 363 lbs (165 kg) and 60 kg/m². *(Bottom)* Eleven months following body lift and 7 months following medial thigh lift with a vertical component.

inconsistent results with regard to scar location, scar quality, and overall outcome. Careful patient marking before a body lift is essential for an optimal outcome. Circumferential body-contouring procedures have the common goal of minimizing scar perceptibility by placing the scar at a level easily concealed by clothing. An analysis of where men and women wear their pants, undergarments, bathing suits, and so forth reveals that the superior portion of most garments in the hip region lies at the level of the

anterior superior iliac spine (ASIS) or approximately 6 to 7 cm below the superior edge of the iliac crest. Posteriorly, garments traverse horizontally

Box 1: Patient selection criteria

- Stable weight
- BMI<35 kg/m²
- Age<55 years
- Hemoglobin ≥ 12

along the lower back and above the buttocks, also at the level of the ASIS. Anteriorly, virtually all undergarments cover the interface between the hair-bearing pubic area and the hypogastrium (Fig. 8). Ideally, the scar for the body lift should be at the level of the ASIS along the hip and lower back and gradually descend to the interface between the hair-bearing pubic area and the hypogastrium anteriorly (see Fig. 8; Fig. 9). An effective technique for marking the body lift should produce a scar that lies reliably along the level of these landmarks, despite the extreme tissue mobility of the patient who has lost a massive amount of weight and the high level of traction required to affect significant change. To do so requires a marking technique that uses bony landmarks, such as the ASIS, to control scar placement.

Preoperative marking

With the patient standing, an area above the buttock cleft is marked first. This point (A), with downward traction to the skin, should be horizontal to the ASIS (see Fig. 9). The ASIS often is difficult to palpate, but is usually at a level approximately three finger breadths (6–7 cm) below the iliac crest. With strong downward traction to the skin along the right anterior iliac region, a point (B) along the anterior axillary line should be marked that is horizontal to point A, also under downward traction (see Fig. 9). A dotted line is drawn from A to B with downward traction over the right thigh and buttock. The dotted line with downward traction should be aligned with the level of the patient's ASIS.

Sitting in front of the patient, the surgeon identifies a symmetric point (C) along the left anterior axillary line. A dotted line is similarly drawn from C to A with downward traction to the left thigh and buttock. With downward traction to the right and left buttocks and thigh areas, a straight dotted line should result from point B on the right to point C on the left, passing through point A over the buttock cleft (see Fig. 9). If the line is straight, the dots are connected.

A point (B′) is identified inferior to point B by the pinch technique. When approximated, the two points eliminate cellulite along the anterior and lateral thigh. A similar procedure is performed on the left side and at the buttock cleft from point A. The redundant skin of the left and right buttocks is estimated with the pinch technique. Points B and B′ and C and C′ are called points of commitment because the surgeon does not remeasure the distance between these points during surgery and commits to removing this skin. The remaining lower set of lines and point A′ are estimates only (see Fig. 9).

The patient is asked to lie supine and flat on the hospital bed. With firm upward traction applied to the redundant skin along the anterior abdominal wall, a transverse line is drawn along the pubic region, D to D′. The line is placed approximately 6 cm superior to the vulvar anterior commissure or base of the penis. Virtually every patient who has lost a large amount of weight has some degree of ptosis and redundancy of the mons pubis following massive weight loss. When marking the lower abdomen in this population, a normal spatial relationship must be restored between the top of the

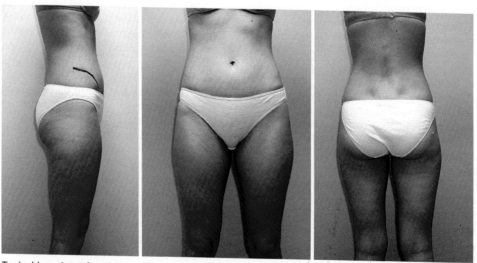

Fig. 8. Typical location of undergarments and their relationship to bony landmarks. Dark line outlines iliac crest. Upper portion of garment lies at level of ASIS.

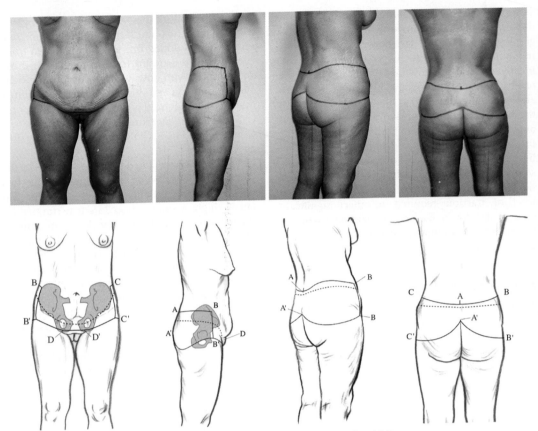

Fig. 9. Body lift marking technique. Dotted line represents where scar should lie.

anterior labial commissure, the top of the hair-bearing pubic area, and the umbilicus. An esthetically pleasing distance from the top of the anterior labial commissure to the top of the hair-bearing pubic area is approximately 6 cm. The umbilicus lies at approximately the level of the iliac crest. If the hair-bearing pubic area were not reduced in the weight loss patient, an esthetically pleasing lower abdomen could not be achieved consistently. With upward traction to the right lower quadrant of the anterior abdominal wall, a straight line is drawn from D to B′, and similarly between D′ and C′, with upward pressure to the left lower quadrant anterior abdominal wall. Traction along the lower quadrants permits correction of some or all of the excess skin along the anterior and medial thighs. In patients who have moderate to severe degrees of skin excess, the lines from D to B′ and D to C′ will lie on the thighs when not on traction.

The patient is asked to stand, and any areas to be liposuctioned are marked at this time.

Intraoperative surgical technique

In the operating room, the patient is prepped with Betadine from the shoulders to the ankles while standing. Then the patient sits on a sterile-draped operating table and is rotated into a supine and flat position. Sterile stockings and sterile sequential compression devices are placed. A draw sheet has been placed previously along the midportion of the table. Following general endotracheal anesthesia, a Foley catheter is placed, and a sterile sheet is stapled to the patient at the level of the inframammary fold and around either flank to nearly the midback. Drapes are placed from the operating table over either arm board. Finally, an ether drape is placed in the usual fashion over the chest area. Grounding pads are placed on each arm and secured with tape.

At the start of the surgical procedure, the skin along the line A to B and A to C is scored superficially. A 1-cm vertical hatch mark is made above point A to demarcate the midline. The skin from B to B′ and from C to C′ and from C′ to B′ across the lower abdomen is incised superficially. If liposuction is to be performed to the thighs, it is done at this time. Full-thickness incisions are made through the skin and soft tissues from C′ to B′ and down to the anterior abdominal wall fascia. The dissection is beveled inferiorly in the region of the mons pubis to directly excise fat in this area, particularly in patients who have higher BMI. Direct excision is more efficient and accurate in this area than is liposuction. Throughout the procedure, the skin is incised with a #10 blade while the subcutaneous tissues are divided and the flaps are elevated with cautery. The cautery is set to a high level. The anterior abdominal wall flap is elevated to the level of the umbilicus, which is preserved in the usual fashion. The skin and underlying subcutaneous tissue along the vertical lines C to C′ and B to B′ are divided to the underlying anterior abdominal wall fascia. Superior to the umbilicus, the dissection is kept primarily over the rectus abdominus muscles to the level of the xiphoid. Every effort is made to preserve intercostal perforators. For patients with more redundant fascia, wider dissection is necessary. The anterior abdominal flap usually is divided along the midline to the level of the umbilicus to allow better exposure of the xiphoid region. The back of the patient is elevated to approximately 35° to further demonstrate fascial laxity. In patients who have had a Lap Band procedure, the port should be addressed at this time. Ports often are secured to the anterior abdominal wall fascia in a paramedian location. With routine plication, the port may be buried and rendered inaccessible. Our approach is to enter the capsule surrounding the port and divide the sutures securing the port to the fascia. The port is then moved to a subcostal position. Plication is then performed, verifying throughout the procedure that the port tube can be moved easily and is not being entrapped by sutures. Once the plication is complete, the port is resecured to the fascia in a subcostal position. To greatly assist in maintaining exposure of the epigastric fascia during plication, a Gomez retractor (Pilling Surgical, Horsham, Pennsylvania) is placed to elevate the anterior abdominal wall flap (Fig. 10). The fascia to be plicated is marked as an ellipse from the pubic bone to the xiphoid. Before plication, 15 mL of 0.25% bupivacaine hydrochloride with 1/200,000 epinephrine is injected into the fascial sheath of each rectus abdominus muscle. Two #1 polypropylene, looped-on sutures (Prolene, Ethicon, Inc., Sommerville, New Jersey) are used to plicate the redundant fascia from the pubic bone to the umbilicus. The two sutures are tied to each other in the midportion of the hypogastric region and buried. The technique avoids the possibility of suture extrusion near incisions or of palpating knots. Two more polypropylene sutures are used to plicate the fascia from the umbilicus to the xiphoid. As the redundant fascia in the epigastric region is plicated, additional undermining of the flap may need to be performed to allow for appropriate contouring.

Then the patient is turned to the left lateral decubital position with assistance from the anesthesiologist behind the ether drape and the use of the draw sheet. With the patient in the left lateral decubital position, the waist is flexed to approximately 30° and the knees to 45°. A full-thickness incision is made in the skin from point B to A and approximately 10 cm beyond A toward C. Incising the skin beyond the midline greatly facilitates undermining in the buttock cleft area and allows for an accurate determination of excess tissue in this region. The skin and subcutaneous tissues are elevated over the right hip, thigh, and buttock. The plane of dissection is made deep to the superficial fascial system in the hip region to include the deep fat compartment. Along the thighs and buttocks, the level of dissection is superficial to the fascia overlying the musculature. The entire deep fat compartment of the hip roll region is removed with this technique, except for some of the fat immediately posterior to the iliac crest. Enough fat should be left behind in this area to prevent an unnatural appearing depression postoperatively. This is particularly important for individuals with higher BMIs. A portion of the deep fat compartment of the hip may lie above the line of incision, but it can be removed along with the flap as it is pulled inferiorly (see Fig. 2; Fig. 11). Liposuction had been performed to the hip roll in the first 50 cases. We found that direct excision of fat was more efficient and precise. Continuous undermining is performed caudally to a level approximately 3 to 4 cm inferior to the line from B′ to A′ except in the buttock cleft region where the undermining is performed only to the level of A′. In the thigh region, continuous undermining is performed to a level just caudal to the greater trochanter. In some women, a 45-cm Lockwood underminer (Byron Medical, Tucson, Arizona) is passed to the knee over the anterior and lateral thigh just superficial to the thigh muscle fascia. The underminer is used on women who demonstrate excess skin and cellulite along the mid and distal one third of the thigh. The waist is flexed to 90° to approximate a sitting position (see Fig. 10). The right lower extremity is abducted to 30° with a Gomez retractor. An abduction pillow maintains the knees approximately 30 cm apart. The right leg is hung by a sterile towel from the Gomez retractor. An Adair clamp is placed between points B and B′, the previously marked points of commitment. A Pitanguy (Padgett Instruments, Kansas City, Missouri) large flap demarcator is used to mark the excess skin along the buttock cleft region. Proper use of the Pitanguy skin marker requires that the clamp be placed in the same plane as the tissues to be measured. If the clamp is off from this plane, the amount of tissue to be excised

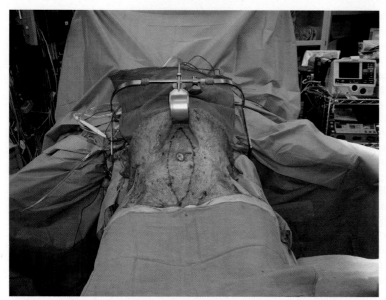

Fig. 10. (*A*) Gomez retractor elevating anterior abdominal wall flap. (*B*) Gomez retractor assisting with patient positioning.

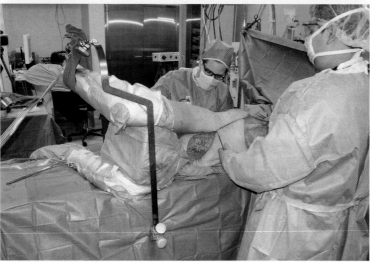

may be overestimated. In measuring with this technique, the amount of traction applied to the flap to be measured is critical. The technique involves securing the Pitanguy marker with an Adair clamp to the flap that has not been undermined and advancing the marker toward the flap to be measured. The nonundermined flap edge usually glides several centimeters before it becomes stable. At this point, the undermined flap is advanced manually into the Pitanguy clamp for measurement. The flap should be advanced toward the clamp until the flap cannot be mobilized any further with moderate tension. Then the tension on the flap is reduced to allow the flap to retract approximately 1 to 2 cm. The flap is marked at that point. The several extra centimeters are important for providing adequate tissue for an optimal closure. The excess skin is

incised, and the point A and a newly established A′ are approximated with an Adair clamp. The tension applied to determine the excess skin at point A is less than at any other point along the wound. With light traction to the right buttock and thigh flap in a cephalic direction, the Pitanguy clamp is used to mark excess skin along these flaps. The excess tissue is removed by incising the skin and beveling the subcutaneous tissues caudally. Normal saline is used to irrigate the thigh and buttock wounds to remove any loose or devitalized tissues. A 10-mm fully perforated flat drain (Zimmer Corp., Dover, Ohio) is placed through a small incision along the lateral aspect of the right side of the pubic area and passed over to the buttock region. The drain is secured in the usual fashion. Adair clamps are used to approximate the upper and lower tissue

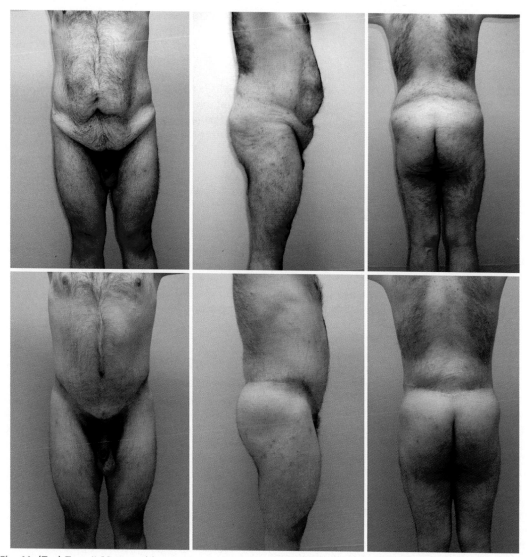

Fig. 11. (*Top*) Type II 33-year-old man 22 months following tubular, banded gastric bypass surgery and weight loss of 155 lbs (70 kg). Current weight and BMI: 200lbs (91 kg) and 30 kg/m², respectively. Maximum weight and BMI: 354 lbs (161 kg) and 52 kg/m², respectively. (*Bottom*) Sixteen months following body lift.

edges of the right buttock and thigh flaps. Number 1 polyglactin 910 (Vicryl, Ethicon, Inc.) stitches are used to approximate the superficial fascial system and deep dermis. 0 polyglactin 910 is placed at the level of the dermis. 3-0 running poliglecaprone 25 (Monocryl, Ethicon, Inc.) is placed at a superficial intracuticular level. The skin is redundant along the closure line and appears as a ridge (Fig. 12). This minimizes tension along the incision during the early months of scar maturation. The patient is turned to the right lateral decubital position, and a similar procedure is performed to the left thigh and buttock. While rotating the patient, Adair clamps are placed at points B–B′ and A–A′ to prevent disruption.

Once in the supine and flat position, the back of the patient is elevated to 35°. Limited undermining of the flap in the epigastric region can lead to flap redundancy and an epigastric roll. For patients with minimal or no lipodystrophy in the epigastric area, this can be addressed by discontinuous undermining digitally or with Mayo scissors opened perpendicularly to the plane of dissection. For some patients, additional undermining may be necessary to eliminate the roll. Every effort is made to preserve intercostal perforators. For patients with an epigastric roll and lipodystrophy in this area, the Pitanguy clamp is used to mark the excess skin at the central portion of the flap. The flap is incised to this point and secured to the lower tissue edge with an Adair

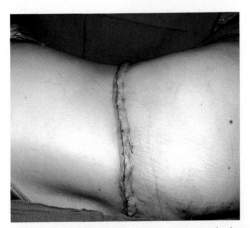

Fig. 12. Appearance of skin edges introperatively as a result of approximation of SFS along with deep dermis.

clamp. Excess flap is marked on either side of the central portion of the flap under slightly more tension than was applied along the midline. Without resecting excess tissue at this time, the flap is secured to the lower tissue edges with additional clamps along the right and left lower quadrants. The patient is returned to a supine and flat position. Liposuction is performed to the epigastric portion of the flap until a roll is no longer present. Following liposuction, the patient's back is elevated once again to 35°. Typically, additional tissue can be marked for excision with the Pitanguy skin marker. Following excision of the excess tissue from the anterior abdominal wall flap, the flap is secured to the lower tissue edge with the patient in a supine and flat position. A new position for the umbilicus is marked, and a 1-cm shield-type incision is made. The umbilical position should be approximately 0.5 cm superior to the corresponding position on the anterior abdominal wall flap to account for the additional retraction that occurs with superficial fascial system (SFS) and deep dermal approximation at the time of closure. The umbilical stalk is secured to the abdominal fascia and dermis of the flap with 3-0 polyglactin 910 sutures. Four additional flat, fully perforated drains are placed through stab wounds in the pubic region. Two of the drains are placed into each thigh recess and two drains onto the abdominal wall fascia. The drains serving the abdominal wall exit the mons pubis medially, and the drains leading to each thigh exit the mons between the drains from each buttock and the abdominal wall. Placing the drains by way of the mons pubis and in a certain order serves several purposes: exiting the drains by way of the mons pubis allows patients to lie comfortably on their back and sides, the preferred positions for patients who have undergone body lifts; the scars from the

drains are less perceptible in the hair-bearing pubic region; not placing the drains along the incision avoids the potential for disruption of the closure; and placing the drains in a specific order and location allows the individual removing the drain to know from which area the drain is being removed. This information can be helpful in preventing seroma formation. The back of the patient is raised to approximately 40°, and the abdominal wall flap is secured to the lower tissue edge as was described for the thigh and buttocks. In addition, the patient also may be placed in a Trendelenburg position to allow the anesthesiologist more access to the airway and to create a more comfortable angle for the surgeon to operate. Interrupted 3-0 polypropylene (Prolene, Ethicon, Inc.) sutures are placed at the umbilicus following approximation with the previously placed 3-0 polyglactin 910 sutures. Sterile dressings are held in place by a loose binder. The patient is transferred to a hospital bed in a beach chair position following extubation.

Optimizing outcomes

Patient classification

Achieving the best results requires a careful assessment and individual approach to each patient. We have found that classifying patients into groups depending on BMI before the body lift to be helpful in this regard. There are several reasons for classifying. The first is to educate patients better on the likelihood of complications. The second is to provide patients with an idea of the expected outcome from the esthetic and functional point of view. Finally, from the plastic surgeon's point of view, classifying patients helps to create a plan for management whether for selection or as an algorithm for treatment. We classify patients into three groups (Box 2). Normal BMI is between 19 and 25 kg/m² (Table 1). We consider our type I patients to be, in effect, normal weight. Typically, with removal of excess skin and soft tissue following a body lift, the patient's BMI decreases to less than 25 kg/m² if it is not already at the time of the body lift (see Fig. 4; Figs 13 and 14). Type II patients usually remain overweight, and type III patients stabilize in the obese category (see Figs. 2, 6, 7, and 11). The approach to each class of patients differs, particularly

Box 2: Patient classification by body mass index
Type I: BMI<28 kg/m²
Type II: 28≤BMI≤32 kg/m²
Type III: BMI>32 kg/m²

Table 1: BMI and obesity	
BMI (kg/m²)	Category
19–24.9	Normal weight
25–29.9	Overweight
30–34.9	Obese
35–39.9	Severely obese
40–49.9	Morbidly obese
50–59.9	Superobese

with regard to the management of lipodystrophy and the sequence of procedures.

Type I patient management (body mass index<28 kg/m²)

Patients with a BMI of less than 28 kg/m² following massive weight loss are the most likely to achieve an ideal body contour and usually have minimal lipodystrophy (see Figs. 4 and 13). Our approach to the lower body in this class of patients is to offer a body lift first (Box 3). Women in this group may have remaining lipodystrophy along the abdomen, hips, and medial and lateral thighs. Excess fat along the hip roll is excised directly, whereas fat along the lateral thighs is liposuctioned. The medial thighs are liposuctioned during the body lift only if the patient is a candidate for and is committed to having a medial thigh lift following the body lift. Liposuction alone to the medial thighs invariably results in skin contour irregularities that can only be addressed with an excisional procedure. Men with a BMI of less than 28 kg/m² following massive weight loss usually have little, if any, lipodystrophy; if they do, it typically is limited to the hip roll or medial thighs. BMI as an indicator of fat content is accurate except in muscular individuals. Men typically have a higher percentage of muscle mass as compared with overall body weight than do women. Men with a BMI of less than 28 kg/m² following massive weight loss, particularly if they are exercising regularly, may appear underweight, but have a BMI that suggests a higher than normal weight. Like woman, excess fat along the hip roll is excised directly in men at the time of the body lift, and fat along the medial thighs is suctioned only if a future medial thigh lift is planned.

Three to 6 months following a body lift, the medial thighs of type I patients are reassessed. The tissue redundancy of the medial thighs is the result of the inferomedial collapse of the excess tissues of the lower abdomen, mons pubis, thighs, and buttocks and the incomplete retraction of the skin and soft tissues of the thighs following massive weight loss. Therefore, the postbariatric thigh deformity is a vertical and horizontal problem. The body lift effectively addresses the vertical component of the medial thigh deformity by the upward and outward rotation of these tissues. The body lift, however, only minimally addresses the horizontal or circumferential thigh deformity by drawing the narrower skin envelope of the distal thigh to the larger proximal thigh. For many type I patients, particularly those younger than 35 years of age or who have a had a BMI change of less than 25 kg/m² following massive weight loss, the body lift may eliminate the need for a formal medial thigh lift (see Fig. 4). Those who are candidates for a medial thigh lift tend to be older or have had a large BMI change (>25–30 kg/m²) following massive weight loss and women with a more gynecoid fat distribution (see Figs. 3 and 5) The appropriate medial lift depends on the remaining thigh deformity following a body lift. In some cases, individuals with excess skin and soft tissue along the proximal medial thigh may be treated effectively with a medial thighplasty limited to the thigh perineal crease. Nevertheless, the addition of a longitudinal component in this group usually produces a better esthetic result with regard to thigh contour and with regard to preventing scar migration from the genitofemoral crease. Patients with a deformity extending to the midthigh or beyond will need a longitudinal component added to their thighplasty. Typically, these individuals have a significant degree of a horizontal deformity or circumferential tissue excess that must be addressed.

Type II patient management (BMI≥28≤32 kg/m²)

Type II patients represent more of a challenge. Lipodystrophy typically is of a much greater concern, particularly for women. Achieving an ideal body contour is less likely for this group. These individuals have a BMI of between 28 and 32 kg/m² and, therefore, are overweight or obese by definition. Following a body lift, they are unlikely to reach a normal BMI and usually stabilize between 25 and 30 kg/m². Liposuction usually plays an important role in thigh management in this group of patients, particularly among women, as does direct excision of fat at the hip region. In general, women in this group, particularly those with a more gynecoid body habitus, are offered a body lift first with extensive outer thigh liposuction (see Fig. 6). Liposuction of the thighs at the time of the body lift addresses lipodystrophy and decreases overall thigh volume, allowing more tissue to be excised vertically. Greater tissue excess may exist circumferentially at the thighs following the body lift and thigh liposuction alone; however, a much more effective thighplasty then can be performed as a second stage. Men and women with a more android body habitus are offered a body lift as well;

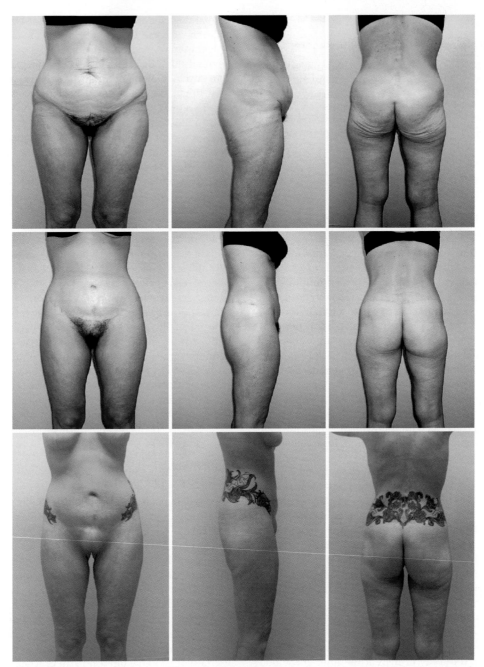

Fig. 13. (*Top*) Type I 46-year-old woman 15 months following tubular, banded gastric bypass surgery and weight loss of 139 lbs (63 kg). Current weight and BMI: 141 lbs (64 kg) and 21 kg/m², respectively. Maximum weight and BMI: 278 lbs (126 kg) and 42 kg/m², respectively. (*Middle*) Two years following body lift. (*Bottom*) Sixty-six months following body lift and additional weight loss of 10 lbs (4.5 kg) over the last 3 years. Note return of some skin excess along thighs.

however, liposuction is performed only along the medial thigh if a medial thigh lift is planned. Direct excision of fat from the hip roll area is important for most type II men and women (see Figs. 6 and 11). As with the type I patients, a medial thigh lift may be necessary following a body lift. The same approach regarding timing and management is used for this heavier group of patients. Repeat liposuction of the thighs is performed often as part of any thighplasty.

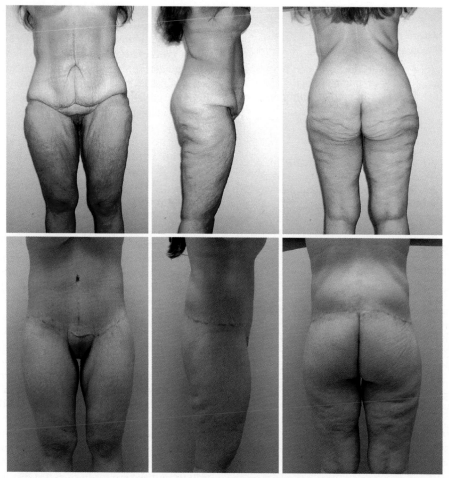

Fig. 14. (*Top*) Type I 42-year-old woman 21 months following tubular banded gastric bypass surgery and weight loss of 153 lbs (70 kg). Current weight and BMI: (71 kg) and 27 kg/m², respectively. Maximum weight and BMI: (141 kg) and 53 kg/m². (*Bottom*) Seven months following full-term pregnancy and 26 months following body lift.

Type III patient management (BMI>32 kg/m²)

Type III patients, those with a BMI of greater than 32 kg/m², are the most challenging. They are the least likely to achieve an ideal body contour. Individuals in this category are obese and are unlikely to fall into the overweight category (BMI 25–30 kg/m²) following plastic surgery. Careful patient selection and staging is particularly important in this group of patients to minimize complications and maximize outcome (see Box 3). Our customary approach to these individuals is as follows. Within the type III category, we separate patients into those with BMI of less than 35 kg/m² and those with BMI greater than 35 kg/m². For men with a BMI of less than 35 kg/m² and age less than 55 years, we offer a body lift first, with possible liposuction of the medial thighs (see Fig. 2). Men older than 55 years of age or with a BMI greater than 35 kg/m² are considered for an abdominoplasty to be followed in 3 to 6 months by a simultaneous thigh and buttock lift as an alternative to the body lift. Women with a BMI of less than 35 kg/m², an android or central distribution of fat, and age less than 55 years are offered a body lift (see Fig. 7) with possible thigh liposuction. Women older than 55 years of age or those with a gynecoid body habitus or a BMI of greater than 35 kg/m² should be considered for an abdominoplasty with thigh liposuction to be followed in 3 to 6 months by a simultaneous thigh and buttock lift (see Fig. 1). Women of this weight and with a gynecoid body habitus typically have a degree of thigh lipodystrophy that would make a primary thigh lifting procedure minimally effective in terms of correcting any distal thigh deformity. Large-volume thigh liposuction at the time of a body lift may increase the morbidity of the procedure significantly, and tissue edema may not permit an accurate assessment of tissue excess. As with the other two categories of patients, type III men and women are

---

Box 3: Patient management

Type I: BMI<28 kg/m²
Men and women

> Body lift + thigh liposuction (medial thighs for men, possibly circumferential in women)
> Evaluate for possible medial thighplasty 3 to 6 months following body lift

Type II: 28≤BMI<32 kg/m²
Men and women

> Body lift + thigh liposuction (medial thighs for men, often circumferential in women)
> Evaluate for possible medial thighplasty 3 to 6 months following body lift

Type III: BMI≥32 kg/m²
Men
BMI<35 kg/m² and age<55 years

> Body lift + medial thigh liposuction

BMI>35 kg/m² or age>55 years

> Consider abdominoplasty with second-stage thigh and buttock lift
> Evaluate for possible medial thighplasty 3 to 6 months following body lift or second stage thigh and buttock lift

Women
BMI<35 kg/m², age<55 years, and android body habitus

> Body lift + thigh liposuction

BMI >35 kg/m², age >55 years, and gynecoid body habitus

> Consider abdominoplasty with thigh liposuction and second-stage thigh and buttock lift
> Evaluate for possible medial thighplasty 3 to 6 months following body lift or second-stage thigh and buttock lift

Avoid medial thigh liposuction with body lift unless future medial thigh lift planned

---

evaluated for a medial thighplasty 3 to 6 months following their final procedure.

Variables affecting esthetic outcome

An assessment of body contour following a body lift demonstrates that the technique produces consistent results when patients of the same gender and similar age, body habitus, BMI, and maximum BMI are compared. For men and women, higher BMI at the time of the body lift and higher maximum BMI before massive weight loss correlate with a lower esthetic outcome. Age and body habitus affect men and women differently, however. Advancing age and gynecoid body habitus in women correlate with a lower esthetic outcome, particularly with regard to remaining skin and cellulite along the distal thighs. In the female patient with a gynecoid body habitus, a significant part of the thigh deformity is the result of a circumferential excess of tissues. The skin of the thighs, particularly in older patients, fails to retract completely to accommodate the smaller volume of the lower extremity. The forces of traction from the body lift originate from the lower torso. As the body contour deformity of the patient who has lost a massive amount of weight extends farther from the lower torso, the effect of the procedures diminishes. The body lift corrects the thigh and buttock deformity of the patient who has lost a massive amount of weight primarily by upward traction and the removal of tissues in this vector; however, the body lift only minimally addresses the circumferential excess of tissues that may be present at the thighs. As a result, older women and women with a more gynecoid body habitus are more likely to have excess skin and cellulite along the distal thighs following a body lift. Conversely, men may be spared entirely of cellulite along the thighs, with most of their excess skin limited to the medial thighs. This seems to be true for older men as well. The deformities of massive weight loss in men are nearly always centered near and around the lower torso (ie, lower abdomen, hips, and proximal medial thighs). This is a direct result of the central or android distribution of fat in men. Consequently, the body lift is consistently effective across a wide range of BMIs and age groups in men. Fat distribution in women is much more variable, with the most common being gynecoid. As would be expected, women with a high BMI who have a more central fat distribution or android body habitus can expect better results from the body lift than can women with a more gynecoid body morphology.

The body lift maintains satisfactory long-term results for patients who minimize sun exposure, do not consume tobacco, and, perhaps most importantly, maintain a steady weight. Weight gain and weight loss can adversely affect esthetic outcome. Weight loss is tolerated well in younger patients in whom some skin elasticity is present. Weight loss in older women can result in a return of cellulite (see Fig. 13). Weight gain can result in a return of lipodystrophy. A cycle of weight gain and loss over years diminishes skin quality. Our routine is to weigh patients during office visits and to remind them of the importance of maintaining a steady weight.

Following weight loss, many young women, particularly those who are eager to have children, are concerned about the potential effects of pregnancy on the long-term outcome of a body lift procedure.

The generally accepted recommendation to women who are considering contouring surgery of the abdomen and who are planning to have children is to forego these procedures until after the birth of their last child. The patient who has lost a massive amount of weight presents a special situation. Many of them have severe contour deformities that impact greatly on their self-esteem. We advise them to postpone having a body lift if they are planning to become pregnant in the near future. If not, we feel comfortable recommending that they proceed with this operation. The cases in which patients have become pregnant following a body lift have revealed that the body contouring results are maintained fairly well (see Fig. 14).

Scar quality

It requires significant tension to affect change along the distal thighs and upper abdomen from the lower torso. Therefore, a properly performed body lift creates the potential for wide and possibly unesthetic scars. During the early part of our body lift series, the SFS was approximated with a braided nylon suture. Then the dermis was approximated as a separate layer with absorbable sutures. Although the soft tissue contour of this group of patients was good over the long-term, the scar quality was variable. Some had wider and more hypertrophic scars than did others. Following the recommendation of Dr. Lockwood (personal communication, 2002), we began incorporating a portion of the dermis with the SFS approximation (see Fig. 12). This modification to our technique allowed us to create some degree of skin redundancy along the closure for as long as 3 months, and, in turn, provided more consistent results with regard to scar quality. Our attempts to create skin redundancy at the incision with approximation of the SFS alone, without the dermis, had been unsuccessful. With this change, we were creating, in effect, a low-tension skin closure with a body contouring procedure incorporating a high level of traction. From this observation, we concluded that although SFS approximation is important for the maintenance of soft tissue contour, minimizing skin tension during the first several months of wound maturation is important to producing satisfactory scars with the body lift. Despite the theoretic advantage of nonabsorbable sutures (braided nylon), permanent suture material has been the cause for several occasional, but recurring, patient complaints. These include suture migration to the skin surface months or even years following the procedure; suture visibility through the skin, particularly in individuals with a fair complexion; and a palpable cord secondary to tension on braided nylon and its surrounding scar capsule in individuals who have gained weight.

Weight gain seems to decrease the overall thickness of the skin, which exacerbates this last patient concern. In an effort to minimize these occasional complaints, we used polyglactin 910 in the last 100 cases. Our reluctance to not use absorbable sutures was based on the concern that suture material with a limited duration in tensile strength may not produce optimum scars. The product insert for polyglactin 910 describes the material as having essentially no tensile strength beyond 5 weeks. We have found that some degree of skin edge eversion remains for approximately 2 months with this material. We do not have long-term results with this suture; however, the scar quality seems comparable to that seen with the braided nylon suture, and this material is unlikely to have any of the other problems associated with permanent suture material.

Postoperative care

Patients are usually restricted to a hospital bed until the next morning. Anticoagulants are not used perioperatively. Sequential compression devices are left in place. Patients are then assisted with ambulation after tolerating a sitting position. The Foley catheter and sequential compression devices are removed if the patient is ambulating well. On postoperative day two, the patient usually is discharged following a lower extremity venous Doppler study. Three postoperative doses of antibiotics are prescribed. Oral narcotics and laxatives are prescribed as well. The first follow-up office visit is 1 week after surgery. At this visit, only drains with an output of less than 30 mL in the previous 24-hour period are removed. At most, two drains are removed at each visit and preferably not from the same side. All drains are removed by 5 weeks, regardless of output. Patients are followed at 6 weeks, 3 months, 6 months, and annually thereafter.

Complications: management and prevention

Complications following the body lift are more frequent than with traditional body-contouring procedures, such as abdominoplasty [4,23,24]. This finding is not surprising considering the much greater magnitude of this procedure and the degree of deformity to be corrected in the population that has lost a massive amount of weight. Nevertheless, complications generally are tolerated well by this patient population because of the often-dramatic functional and esthetic benefits that come with these procedures. The overall complication rate for the first 425 body lifts in our experience was 49.7% (Table 2). Statistical analysis of the data revealed that patients with higher maximum BMIs before massive weight loss are at a greater risk for complications following a body lift ($P<.01$). For

Table 2: Patient outcome data

Cases	N (%)	LOS (d)	Drain duration (d)	Complications (%)	Dehiscence (%)	Seroma (%)	Skin necrosis (%)	Infection (%)	Bleeding (%)	DVT (%)	PE (%)	Transfusions (%)
Total	425* (100.00)	2.74	23	49.65	27.29	20.94	8.47	4.94	2.59	2.35	1.18	12.94
Women	361 (84.94)	2.70	22	40.94	27.42	18.56	9.14	4.99	2.22	2.22	1.39	11.91
Men	64 (15.06)	2.98	27	57.81	26.56	34.38	4.69	4.69	4.69	3.13	0.00	18.75
Type 1	207 (48.71)	2.44	21	44.44	25.60	16.91	10.14	3.86	1.45	0.97	0.00	8.21
Type 2	126 (29.65)	2.84	25	51.59	26.98	26.19	5.56	3.17	3.97	3.97	1.59	15.87
Type 3	92 (21.65)	3.29	25	58.70	31.52	22.83	8.70	9.78	3.26	3.26	3.26	19.57
Nonsmokers	363 (85.41)	2.75	23	47.93	26.17	19.83	7.44	5.51	3.03	2.75	1.38	14.05
Type 1	172 (83.09)	2.35	22	41.86	25.00	15.70	6.98	4.07	1.74	1.16	0.00	8.14
Type 2	110 (87.30)	2.92	25	50.91	25.45	26.36	6.36	3.64	4.55	4.55	1.82	17.27
Type 3	81 (88.04)	3.37	25	56.79	29.63	19.75	9.88	11.11	3.70	3.70	3.70	22.22
Smokers	62 (14.59)	2.68	21	59.68	33.87	27.42	14.52	1.61	0.00	0.00	0.00	6.45
Type 1	35 (16.91)	2.91	20	57.14	28.57	22.86	25.71	2.86	0.00	0.00	0.00	8.57
Type 2	16 (12.70)	2.31	22	56.25	37.50	25.00	0.00	0.00	0.00	0.00	0.00	6.25
Type 3	11 (11.96)	2.73	24	72.73	45.45	45.45	0.00	0.00	0.00	0.00	0.00	0.00

Abbreviations: DVT, deep vein thrombosis; LOS, length of stay; PE, pulmonary embolism.
* Simultaneous abdominoplasty and thigh and buttock lift (body lift).

example, an individual with a maximum BMI of 70 kg/m^2 before massive weight loss has a 15 times greater chance of having complications following a body lift than does somebody with a BMI of 40 kg/m^2. Patients with larger changes in BMI after weight loss also are at greater risk for complications ($P<.03$). Although type III patients (BMI>32 kg/m^2) had more complications than did type I individuals (BMI<28 kg/m^2), BMI at the time of the body lift did not have a significant association with complications ($P<.1$). Patients with a history of smoking had a significantly greater risk for complications ($P<.01$), including skin dehiscence and skin necrosis. Men had a higher complication rate than did women; however, the association with gender was not significant ($P<.1$). Age at the time of the body lift also was not correlated significantly with complications.

Skin dehiscence

In our experience, skin dehiscence is the most frequent complication following a body lift (see Table 2). This can be attributed to the fact that the procedure is circumferential and that a high degree of traction is needed to produce an ideal outcome. Nevertheless, the frequency and severity of this complication has continued to diminish, particularly in the last 50 cases. In most cases in our series, skin dehiscence has occurred at the buttock cleft and hips—the two areas of greatest tension following this procedure. In the early part of the series, the skin to be removed at the buttock cleft was measured with the patient standing before surgery. During surgery, the waist was not flexed completely into a sitting position, and the previously marked skin to be removed appeared to be appropriate. Assuming a sitting position places significant tension on this minimally mobile part of the lower back. In addition, the greater period of time in bed in the early postoperative period may lead to some degree of ischemia over the sacrum and coccyx, likely contributing to poor healing in this area. Measuring the tissue to be removed intraoperatively, with the patient flexed into a sitting position, has greatly decreased the frequency and severity of this problem. In the last 50 cases, we have limited the direct undermining in the buttock cleft region to the lower line of resection. This has increased the vascularity of the lower flap and helped to diminish the incidence of skin dehiscense. The hip had been another problem area for skin dehiscence in the early part of our series. Approximating the SFS along with a small dermal component, as suggested by Lockwood, allowed us to create some degree of tissue redundancy along the closure for several months. We believe that this modification to our technique decreased the incidence of skin dehiscence and improved scar quality. Most of skin dehiscences in our experience have been 1 to 2 cm in length and occurred more than 2 weeks following surgery. We have not had an acute skin dehiscence in over 200 cases. The vast majority of skin dehiscences reported in this series are secondary to poor healing and diminished blood supply (ie, marginal ischemia). These dehiscences have been managed successfully with local wound care. The few acute dehiscences were managed surgically. In six cases, nonabsorbable stitches were placed at the bedside on postoperative day one or two to approximate skin edges. In two other instances, patients fainted while showering for the first time, leading to a large wound dehiscence and an immediate return to the operating room. We now advise patients to take their first shower following surgery with assistance and close supervision. The key elements to preventing skin dehiscence are an effective and reliable preoperative marking technique, accurate intraoperative tissue measurement, and a closure technique that minimizes tension along the skin edges in the postoperative period.

Seroma

Seroma formation remains a frequent complication following body lifts in the postbariatric population. Extensive tissue undermining and the shearing of opposing subcutaneous tissue surfaces predispose patients to this complication. The reported incidence of seromas varies significantly in the literature, as does the approach to their prevention. Aly and colleagues [5] reported a rate of 37.5% and described removing all drains by 2 weeks. Carwell and Horton [9] and Van Geertruyden and colleagues [7] described seroma rates of 14% and 6.6%, respectively. In a series of 40 cases, Pascal and Le Louarn [11] reported no seromas and removed all drains by 3 days postoperatively. In our series of 425 cases, we had a seroma rate of 20.9%, with the last drain removed after an average of 23 days (see Table 2). All seromas involved the thigh, and, in some cases, extended to the buttocks or the anterior abdominal wall. The explanation for the pattern of seromas at the thigh most likely has to do with the motion of the greater trochanter with ambulation and this being the most dependent area of continuous undermining. In our technique, the drains are placed through the mons pubis in a specific order and to a designated location. Our usual practice is to begin removing drains 1 week following surgery. Typically, the two drains serving the abdomen are removed first. The drains are removed only if they are draining less than 30 mL in a 24-hour period. The following week, the drains servicing each thigh recess are removed, and the buttock drains are removed at approximately 3 weeks. The buttock drains treat the thigh recess as well. Any remaining drain is removed at 5 weeks, regardless of output. Knowing where each drain is placed eliminates the possibility of removing two drains from the same side of the body. At each office visit, the drains are stripped to verify patency and proper function. We believe that this is important, particularly in patients who may have had some oozing in the immediate postoperative period. Frequently, a drain that appears to be ready to be removed may be obstructed by coagulated blood or fibrin. Our initial approach to seromas is to drain the collection by needle aspiration. If the patient presents with any signs or symptoms of infection or the quality of the fluid suggests infection, the fluid is sent for analysis, and a 10-mm fully perforated flat drain is placed into the seroma cavity by way of the body lift scar. If the seroma is larger than 10 cm in diameter and clinically sterile, the patient is offered the possibility of having a drain placed in the cavity. Anther option is to place a Penrose drain into the seroma cavity by way of the scar. We have used this latter technique on two occasions, both successfully. For patients having to travel long distances for office visits, a standard drain or Penrose drain may represent the better option. Seroma formation can be kept to a reasonably low level by keeping to a carefully prescribed drain protocol and meticulous drain care.

Skin necrosis

In our experience, the most frequent sites for skin necrosis have been the suprapubic region and, less commonly, the hips and buttock cleft. Skin necrosis in body-contouring surgery usually is the result of poor tissue circulation, which can be influenced by variables such as tension, tobacco consumption, scars, liposuction, and, in certain instances, pressure from dressings and garments [24–26]. Necrosis along the suprapubic portion of the abdominal wall flap can be explained readily by the random and peripheral origin of its blood supply following an abdominoplasty. The necrosis along the hips and buttock cleft usually is marginal in presentation and may have more to do with the effect of tension on tissue perfusion. In an effort to preserve the blood supply to the hypogastric portion of the abdominal wall flap, we limit undermining at the epigastrium as much as possible. This concept has been described well [18]. Tissue redundancy in the epigastrium may result from this technique. Liposuction or discontinuous undermining can treat this contour tissue effectively. We prefer to excise any excess fat in the hypogastric portion of the flap. This is performed with curved Mayo scissors and is limited to the fat deep to Scarpa's fascia. The avoidance of liposuction to the infraumbilical

portion of the flap has been advocated by other investigators [23]. Our approach to the prevention of marginal skin necrosis at the hips is to apply only minimal tension to the thigh and buttock flap when measuring for excision and to limit direct undermining to only a few centimeters beyond the tissue to be excised. Because the thigh is abducted when the tissues are being measured, even minimal tension results in significant tension along the lateral thigh when adducted. Anecdotally, we have never seen an esthetic or functional benefit, in terms of preventing complications, from the use of abdominal or thigh garments; however, early in our experience with the body lift, we had two instances in which a netting used to hold dressings in place rolled into a cord, producing a tourniquet effect on the lower abdomen and subsequent skin necrosis. Therefore, because of the potential for garments to diminish circulation, particularly to the lower abdomen, we use only a loosely placed binder in the perioperative period to secure dressings. After 48 hours, when the dressings are removed, patients are advised that they may remove the binder and if they choose to continue to use it, it should be placed loosely. Our necrosis rate is higher than reported by other investigators (see Table 2) [5,7,9,11]. We can attribute this to the fact that 14.6% of our patients have a history of smoking. Tobacco consumption is a well-known appetite suppressant and, not surprisingly, smokers are overrepresented in our patients with the lowest BMIs (Table 3). Although all of our patients are advised not to consume tobacco during the perioperative period, we suspect that some smokers only diminish tobacco consumption during that time. We continue to operate on individuals with a history of tobacco consumption after careful patient education and selection, because the functional and esthetic benefits have outweighed sequelae from skin-healing problems. Upper abdominal scars, particularly those in the right and left subcostal region, represent a risk factor for skin necrosis along the lower abdomen. Our approach to patients with these scars is to proceed with the abdominoplasty portion of the operation as described above, with careful attention to minimizing dissection in the epigastric region. The portion of the flap inferior to the flap is monitored carefully. If the lower portion of the flap appears viable, in nearly all instances, we have completed the procedure as usual with no adverse sequelae. If there is concern for the viability of the flap during the procedure, the ischemic area may be excised in a fashion similar to a fleur-de-lis procedure. Most cases of skin necrosis in our series were 1 or 2 cm in greatest diameter and, in all instances, were treated with sharp debridement or dressing changes. Patients are advised

Table 3: Patient characteristics

Cases	N (%)	Maximum BMI (kg/m²)	Current BMI (kg/m²)	BMI Change (kg/m²)	Smokers (%)	Diabetes (%)	HTN (%)
Total	425 (100.00)	50	29	21	14.59	3.06	6.82
Women	361 (84.94)	49	28	20	15.51	3.05	6.37
Men	64 (15.06)	56	32	24	9.38	3.13	9.38
Type 1	207 (48.71)	45	25	20	16.91	2.42	1.93
Type 2	126 (29.65)	50	30	21	12.70	3.97	11.11
Type 3	92 (21.65)	58	35	23	11.96	3.26	11.96
Nonsmokers	363 (85.41)	50	29	21	0	3.03	6.61
Type 1	172 (83.09)	45	25	20	0	2.33	1.74
Type 2	110 (87.30)	51	30	21	0	3.64	10.91
Type 3	81 (88.04)	58	35	23	0	3.70	11.11
Smokers	62 (14.59)	49	28	21	100.00	3.23	8.06
Type 1	35 (16.91)	45	25	20	100.00	2.86	2.86
Type 2	16 (12.70)	49	30	20	100.00	6.25	12.50
Type 3	11 (11.96)	62	36	26	100.00	0.00	18.18

Abbreviation: HTN, hypertension.

that scars from skin necrosis can be evaluated for revision at 1 year postoperatively. Skin necrosis can be minimized by the judicious use of continuous dissection and liposuction in the epigastric region, appropriate use of tension when marking for tissue excision, and the avoidance of garments that may affect circulation, particularly in the early postoperative period. Individuals with a history of tobacco consumption may be eliminated as candidates for a body lift or considered on a case-by-case basis after careful and detailed education.

Infection

Infections have been an infrequent problem in our series (see Table 2). We describe infections as cases in which surgical intervention was required to drain a collection or abscess. We have not had a case of cellulitis without a collection. In nearly all cases, the infections in our series seemed to be seromas-that were clinically evident or undiagnosed and became infected. Collections were treated with open drainage or open drainage with replacement of a 10-mm fully perforated flat drain in the collection cavity. The drainage was sent for analysis, and the patients were placed on oral or intravenous antibiotics. The pathogenesis of infected seromas is unclear. A possibility includes bacteria tracking from the skin on drains and infecting devitalized tissue, probably fat. Drains kept for long periods of time may create a risk factor for this problem. Our previous protocol had been to keep patients on antibiotics until the last drain was removed. This extended antibiotic regimen may predispose patients to infections with more resistant organisms. We now give a single preoperative dose of antibiotics and three postoperative dosages [27].

Hematoma/bleeding

Bleeding and blood loss during and following body lifts is a major concern. Many aspects of these procedures predispose patients to a risk for blood loss. To effectively treat the lower body contour deformity of the patient who has lost a massive amount of weight requires extensive tissue undermining and, with that, the need to ligate or cauterize a multitude of blood vessels. Meticulous hemostasis is critical throughout these procedures. We have found cautery set to a high level to be helpful in this regard. Heavier patients, men, and those with larger BMI changes are at greater risk for significant blood loss. We avoid the routine use of anticoagulants in the perioperative period because of the concern for bleeding. Following malabsorptive bariatric procedures, menstruating women often present with significant degrees of anemia. All patients who have undergone bariatric surgery are advised to take iron supplements when considering body-contouring surgery, and those with more severe cases of anemia are referred to a hematologist. We avoid having an already anemic patient bank autologous blood in the 1-month period before a body lift. Rather, we prefer to transfuse nonautologous blood if it becomes necessary. Our transfusion rate has decreased slightly over the course of the series. Our hematoma rate has remained low at 2.6% (see Table 2). We defined a hematoma as a collection of blood that required surgery for evacuation. We presume that there may be other, smaller hematomas that go unnoticed or are evacuated by the drains themselves.

Deep vein thrombosis and pulmonary embolism

Deep vein thrombosis and pulmonary embolism represent the most serious risk for patients who undergo body lifts. Several recognized risk factors for deep vein thrombosis are fundamental to these procedures [28]. On average, the population of patients are overweight (see Table 3), and the body lift is a lengthy procedure. To complicate matters further, early ambulation can be difficult, and the early, routine use of anticoagulants may create a significant risk for bleeding. Our approach to the avoidance of deep vein thrombosis is to provide continuous mechanical anticoagulation until the patient is ambulatory. Patients are kept on bed rest until the day following surgery. A lower extremity venous Doppler is obtained on the day of discharge. Our deep vein thrombosis rate is 2.4%. We would expect this number to be significantly lower if all of our patients were not studied routinely. Pulmonary embolism remains rare in our series. The management of this life-threatening complication in the patient who has undergone a body lift presents special challenges. Heparinization of the early postoperative patient may lead to significant bleeding. The timing and dosing of heparin must be evaluated carefully as should the possible need for a vena caval filter.

Sequence and combinations of procedures

Individuals who have lost massive amounts of weight often are candidates for, and are eager to have, multiple procedures. Initially, younger patients tend to present with more concerns about their torso and breasts, whereas older patients often have issue with their face and arms. The medial thighs and flanks can be of primary concern for both groups. Our preference regarding the torso is to perform a body lift first, as a single procedure. The body lift may eliminate the need for a formal medial thigh lift in many patients, particularly those younger than 35 years of age and who have had a BMI change of less than 20 to 25 kg/m^2 before the body lift. Furthermore, a more effective medial thigh lift can be performed in a patient following a body lift. The forces of traction of a body lift and medial thigh lift performed concomitantly are usually in opposite directions and are likely to compromise the outcome of one or both procedures [29]. The body lift often can have a significant effect on the upper body (ie, breasts, flanks, and back) (see Figs. 6 and 7). In men, it may eliminate the need for upper body-contouring surgery or reduce the magnitude of the procedure required. In women, although the body lift can impact the back and flanks positively, it also can cause significant downward migration of the inframammary fold. For this reason, ideally, we prefer not to perform breast surgery before or concomitantly with a body lift. Following a body lift, we commonly perform other body-contouring procedures, including combination brachioplasty and mammoplasty, thighplasty alone, or thighplasty with brachioplasty; in certain individuals we perform a combination of the three procedures.

Summary

The body in the patient who has lost a massive amount of weight presents an extreme form of traditional esthetic and functional body contour concerns. Routine body-contouring procedures usually produce only suboptimal results in this patient population. The body lift described above is an excellent alternative to treat the body deformity of the patient who has undergone bariatric surgery. As with every technique, careful patient selection, education, and preparation are critical to minimizing complications and optimizing outcome.

References

[1] Capella JF. Approach to the lower body after weight loss. In: Rubin JP, Matarasso A, editors. Aesthetic surgery after massive weight loss. Philadelphia: Elsevier; 2007. p. 69–99.

[2] Capella JF, Capella RF. Bariatric surgery in adolescence. Is this the best time to operate? Obes Surg 2003;13:826–32.

[3] Capella JF, Capella RF. An assessment of vertical banded gastroplasty-Roux-en-Y gastric bypass for the treatment of morbid obesity. Am J Surg 2002;183:117–23.

[4] Capella JF, Oliak DA, Nemerofsky RB. Body lift: an account of 200 consecutive cases in the massive weight loss patient. Plast Reconstr Surg 2006;117:414.

[5] Aly AS, Cram AE, Chao M, et al. Belt lipectomy for circumferential truncal excess: The University of Iowa experience. Plast Reconstr Surg 2003;111: 398–413.

[6] Lockwood TE. Lower-body lift. Aesthetic Surg J 2001;21:355–70.

[7] Van Geertruyden JP, Vandeweyer E, de Fontaine S, et al. Circumferential torsoplasty. Br J Plast Surg 1999;52:623–8.

[8] Mallory GN. American Society for Bariatric Surgery. Membership survey, 2004.

[9] Carwell GR, Horton CE. Circumferential torsoplasty. Ann Plast Surg 1997;38:213–6.

[10] Hurwitz DJ. Single-staged total body lift after massive weight loss. Ann Plast Surg 2004;52: 435–41.

[11] Pascal JF, Le Louarn C. Remodeling bodylift with high lateral tension. Aesthetic Plast Surg 2002;26: 223–30.

[12] Hamra ST. Circumferential body lift. Aesthetic Surg J 1999;19:244–51.

[13] Morales Gracia HJ. Circular lipectomy with lateral thigh-buttock lift. Aesthetic Plast Surg 2003;27:50.

[14] Regnault P, Daniel R. Secondary thigh-buttock deformities after classical techniques: prevention and treatment. Clin Plast Surg 1984;11: 505–16.

[15] Lockwood TE. Fascial anchoring technique in medial thigh lifts. Plast Reconstr Surg 1988;82: 299–304.

[16] Lockwood T. Superficial fascial system (SFS) of the trunk and extremities: a new concept. Plast Reconstr Surg 1991;87:1009–27.

[17] Lockwood T. Transverse flank-thigh-buttock lift with superficial fascial suspension. Plast Reconstr Surg 1993;92:1112–22.

[18] Lockwood T. High-lateral-tension abdominoplasty with superficial fascial suspension. Plast Reconstr Surg 1995;96:603–15.

[19] Marceau S, Hould FS, Simard S, et al. Biliopancreatic diversion with duodenal switch. World J Surg 1998;22:947–54.

[20] Chapman AE, Kiroff G, Game P, et al. Laparoscopic adjustable gastric banding in the treatment of obesity: a systematic literature review. Surgery 2004;135:326–51.

[21] Capella JF, Capella RF. The weight reduction operation of choice: vertical banded gastroplasty or gastric bypass? Am J Surg 1996;171:74–9.

[22] Brolin RE. Metabolic deficiencies and supplements following bariatric operations. In: Martin L, editor. Obesity surgery. New York: McGraw-Hill; 2004. p. 275–300.

[23] Matarasso A. Liposuction as an adjunct to a full abdominoplasty. Plast Reconstr Surg 1995;95: 829–36.

[24] Chaouat M, Levan P, Lalanne B, et al. Abdominal dermolipectomies: early postoperative complications and long-term unfavorable results. Plast Reconstr Surg 2000;106:1614–23.

[25] El-khatib HA, Bener A. Abdominal dermolipectomy in an abdomen with pre-existing scars: a different concept. Plast Reconstr Surg 2004; 114:992–7.

[26] Manassa EH, Hertl CH, Olbrisch R. Wound healing problems in smokers and nonsmokers after 132 abdominoplasties. Plast Reconstr Surg 2003;111:2082–7.

[27] Barie PS. Surgical site infections: epidemiology and prevention. Surgical infections 2002;3:S9–20.

[28] Geerts WH, Heit JA, Clagett GP, et al. Prevention of venous thromboembolism. Chest 2001;119: 132S–75S.

[29] Aly AS, Capella JF. Staging, reoperation, and treatment of complications after body contouring in the massive-weight-loss patient. In: Grotting JC, editor. Reoperative aesthetic and reconstructive plastic surgery. 2nd edition. St. Louis (MO): Quality Medical Publishing; 2007. p. 1701–40.

ELSEVIER
SAUNDERS

CLINICS IN
PLASTIC
SURGERY

Clin Plastic Surg 35 (2008) 53–71

Circumferential Lower Truncal Dermatolipectomy

Dirk F. Richter, MD*, Alexander Stoff, MD,
Fernando J. Velasco-Laguardia, MD,
Matthias A. Reichenberger, MD

The increase of obesity and overweight in the general population has stimulated many approaches to treat this condition from a clinical perspective. In addition to the multitude of surgical measures for reducing weight, a large number of conservative treatment procedures, such as diets, nutritional substitutes, psychotherapy, acupuncture, and monitoring procedures, have been developed. In addition to gastroscopically inserted gastric balloons, numerous other procedures for reducing the stomach size, performing a gastric bypass, or gastric banding have been established. Since its inception in 1966, bariatric sugery has offered the greatest degree of sustained weight loss to morbidly obese [1,2].

Because of the alarming increase in obesity in the general population, as well as the increasingly improved surgical and conservative measures that have become available for controlling overweight, the number of patients with a history of extreme overweight and weight loss has increased significantly over the last several years. In the present authors' own patient group, weight reductions of up to 210 kg have been observed. Congruent with this has been the problem of surplus and overhanging skin, which has also become more evident and frequent. Skin-lifting operations available until now (eg, abdominal lipectomy, thigh and buttock lifting) have often fallen short of producing an aesthetically acceptable overall outcome.

Following the establishment of modern body lift procedures by Ted Lockwood, who, sadly, passed away in 2005, other innovative approaches are also now available. The main idea behind these

Department of Plastic and Reconstructive Surgery, Dreifaltigkeits-Hospital, Bonner Strasse 84, 50389 Wesseling, Germany
* Corresponding author.
E-mail address: Dr.Dirk.Richter@t-online.de (D.F. Richter).

doi:10.1016/j.cps.2007.09.001
plasticsurgery.theclinics.com

operations, similar to modern facelift procedures, is to reconstruct the superficial and deep connective tissue layers comparable to the superficial musculoaponeurotic system (SMAS) of the face. Large-area tissue undermining and separation are, however, necessary to allow sufficient mobilization and tightening of the affected areas.

At the same time, it must be remembered that patients who have undergone major weight loss often have intrinsic medical problems such as diabetes mellitus, high blood pressure, nicotine abuse, and hormonal derailment. These factors must be considered when planning the reconstruction of the body contour if problems are to be avoided.

The problems and solutions discussed in this article derive from the experience collected over the last 10 years at the Department of Plastic and Reconstructive Surgery at the Dreifaltigkeits-Hospital in Wesseling, Germany. These surgical procedures are the operations with the largest treated body surface area with manageable risks when the planning and operation are performed meticulously and conscientiously [3].

Overview

With surgical reconstruction after severe weight loss, conventional corrective procedures such as thigh and buttock lift are often stretched to their limits. "Dog-ears," unsightly scars, or flattening of body curves may occur. Because of these limitations, circumferential lift procedures have been further developed since the 1960s, including (1) circumferential abdominal lipectomy, (2) belt lipectomy, (3) lower body lift, and (4) circumferential suprafascial lower trunk dermatolipectomy.

Circumferential abdominal lipectomy

A circumferential abdominal lipectomy is defined as an abdominoplasty with an incision course that extends into the area of the back and buttocks. It serves solely to prevent dog-ears and exerts no tightening effect on the back or buttocks. It produces much scarring with unsatisfactory results in dorsal areas (Fig. 1).

Belt lipectomy

The belt lipectomy, described by Gonzales-Uloa [4] and modified by Aly [5], represents a much more extensive surgical procedure with its own philosophy. In this operation, a circumferential wedge of tissue in the shape of a belt is excised that is more extensive and broader compared with the circumferential abdominal lipectomy. The resection occurs directly at the problematic areas of surplus tissue at the hip and back, and leaves a circumferential scar in the area of the waist above the iliac crest. These

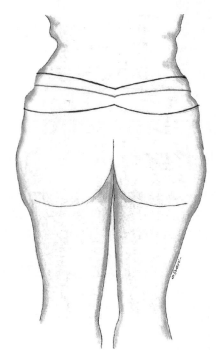

Fig. 1. Posterior markings for the circumferential abdominal lipectomy. Blue markings indicate the upper and lower incision lines and red marking indicates the resulting scar line.

often relatively high scars are consciously weighed against the benefit of the improved accentuation of the figure, particularly in the waist area. Because of the height of the scar, tightening at the back is excellent. The "tent shape" effect typical for the body lift that arises from the downward pulling of the soft-tissue flap of the back is not observed here (Fig. 2).

Lower body lift

In 1993 Lockwood provided a key contribution to body lift operations with his lower body lift. This approach is a thigh-truncal lift that intentionally eliminates the lateral and anterolateral zones of adherence, which helps to promote a pull from the knee up. The meticulous handling of the zones of adherence and the superficial fascia system (SFS) led to a new, integrated concept that is of particular importance for patients who have undergone severe weight loss [6–8].

Over the last few years, experience has been gained with more than 500 patients, initially with the Lockwood lower body lift and the belt lipectomy, and then with modifications of these as well as other entirely different concepts [5,9–15].

Lockwood dissected below the scarpa fascia, which resulted in a complete suprafascial (above the fascia) soft-tissue layer being resected. This led to a volume

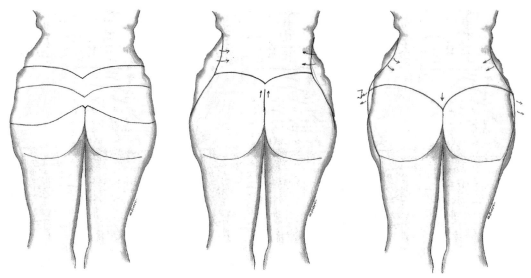

Fig. 2. Posterior markings for belt lipectomy (*left*). Blue markings indicate the upper and lower incision lines and red marking indicates the resulting scar line. Superior waist form improvement after belt lipectomy (*center*) compared with lower body lift (*right*).

reduction, particularly in the area of the buttocks, which in turn resulted in a flattening of the buttocks. In addition, no real three-dimensional tightening was possible through a reconstruction of the scarpa fascia at the height of the skin incision, as the direction of the tension vectors from the skin and fascia sutures extends in the same direction (Fig. 3).

The present authors' approach of a circumferential suprafascial dermatolipectomy differs in several respects (Box 1).

In regard to the authors' technique, three possible variations have been identified: original technique, modified technique, and combination technique. In all three variations the dorsal

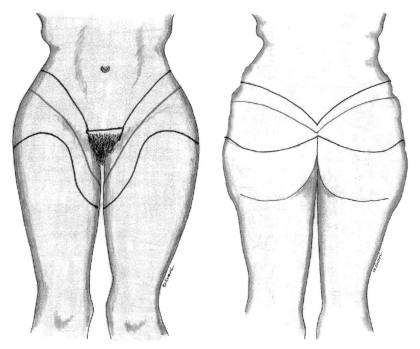

Fig. 3. Anterior (*left*) and posterior (*right*) markings for the body lift, inaugurated by Ted Lockwood. Blue markings indicate the upper and lower incision lines and red marking indicates the resulting scar line.

1. Dissection occurs suprafascially, whether dorsally or ventrally up to the umbilicus. The stronger and denser superficial fat can then be spared and used for the volume reconstruction dorsally. The fascia remains attached to the deep fat, in the area of resection circumferentially. Because of this the resilient fascia can be used for repositioning and remodeling in different vectors in relation to the skin. Regularly, the hip and gluteal fat falls laterally to the waist when the patient is in the prone position. Here, the fascia can be satisfactorily grasped on the side with a robust, non-resorbable suture and medially repositioned. A satisfactory engorgement of the superficial and deep fat tissue results, so that the maximal projections lie in the upper portions of the buttocks. Replacing the mobilized skin above this reconstructed area produces a satisfactory volume redistribution. In the area not to be resected, the superficial fascia remains conformant with the skin, so that any additional tension can be absorbed when performing the final suturing (Figs. 4 and 5).
2. The stretching of the superficial fascia system occurs in the vertical-medial direction independently of the vector along which the skin is stretched. This allows a three-dimensional, bi-vectoral reconstruction of the buttocks, hips, and waist. In addition, the superficial fascia reconstruction in the area of the buttocks absorbs much of the tension. This effect is referred to as the "gluteal superficial musculoaponeurotic system," analogous to the same principle applied with modern facelifts (Fig. 6).
3. In the area of the abdomen, resection is first performed suprafascially until three-finger breadth below the umbilicus. This ensures that the lymph drainage pathways that are plentiful in this region remain unscathed. Also, strongly pulling the fascia achieves an additional lifting effect on the thighs and the mons pubis. Scarpa's fascia is then affixed to the superficial rectus muscle fascia at approximately the height of the umbilicus using robust, non-resorbable suture material. It is important to break through Scarpa's fascia down to the anterior rectus fascia below the upper resection line. Doing so prevents the suprafascial vascular plexus—and the blood supply associated with it—from being destroyed cranially, and Scarpa's fascia can be adapted before closure of the skin (Fig. 7).

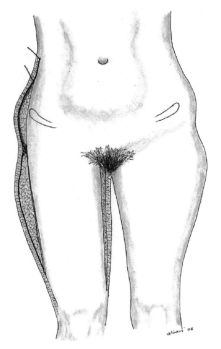

Fig. 4. Front view demonstration of the different lateral dissection levels (*red line*). Above the height of the gluteal fold the dissection is performed suprafascially, whereas the level below changes further deep to the epimusculofascial plane after detachment of the lateral adherences (zones of adherence).

markings do not differ, but the ventral markings do [3,8,12,16].

Markings

Initially, the boundaries of the patient's undergarments are marked while the patient is standing. The patient is asked to wear a preferred undergarment that is not too tight, which will cover scars that are not susceptible to any "fashion-related" changes (eg, high-cut bikini versus deep-set hip jeans). The desired scar line is marked in red after consulting with the patient. Markings of the back are identical with all three variations of the technique, and they are performed first (Fig. 8).

The posterior upper incision line runs about two- to three-finger breadth above the planned scar line and is marked in blue. The blue line, along its entire length, is then pulled down using the examiner's palm and is checked to make sure that it will reach the proposed red line of closure. The inferior proposed line of excision is estimated by strongly pinching the skin below the red line dorsally and laterally, ensuring that approximately a quarter of the total resection height lies superior to the red scar line while the lower three quarters

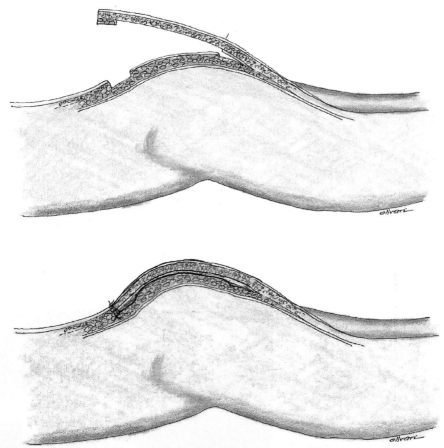

Fig. 5. Lateral view demonstration of the different gluteal dissection levels after dissection (*top*) and after wound closure (*bottom*). From the initially suprafascial plane the cut is made through the superficial fascia at the height of the tronchanter and continues undermining subfascially before descending laterally to the level above the tensor muscle fascia.

are inferior to it. The inferior proposed line of excision is an estimate that may need to be adjusted at the time of surgery. The rima ani should not be elevated if avoidable, as an excessively long gluteal furrow may otherwise result. It has been worthwhile to allow the upper incision line to run a little more sharply angled into the gluteal furrow, to also achieve an optical accentuation of the buttock form (see Fig. 8; Fig. 9). Next, the anterior markings are performed based on the frontal red line previously marked.

With the original technique, the marking first begins with a steep rising vertical line parallel to the lateral boundary of the mons pubis, which is then continued at the height of the umbilicus in a steep curved course to the upper horizontal dorso-lateral line. According to the back markings, the upper and lower incision lines are adjusted to the marked anticipated scar line, considering the vertical ratio of one quarter of tissue above and three quarters below this line. The steeper the rising line is formed, the better the caudo-lateral stretching effect at the upper abdomen. The "pinch test" is once again essential for the lower incision line, which then runs parallel and tightly alongside the scar and upper incision line at the height of the mons pubis. In case of a required inner thigh lift, the upper incision line is then started slightly above the inguinal fold, which terminates at the end of the labia majora without continuing dorsally. Then the lower incision line is marked, which must be pinched out carefully. If a sagging mons pubis and/or a moderate vertical lower abdominal slackening is evident, a horizontal incision line can be marked slightly above the mons pubis (see Fig. 3).

The modified technique resembles the marking of a conventional abdominoplasty, except that the lateral upper incision line continues to the back region without the ends tapering to a lateral point. The ratio between the vertical abdominal resection area above and below the resulting scar line is 4:1 (Fig. 10). Frequently, the resulting scar line is placed

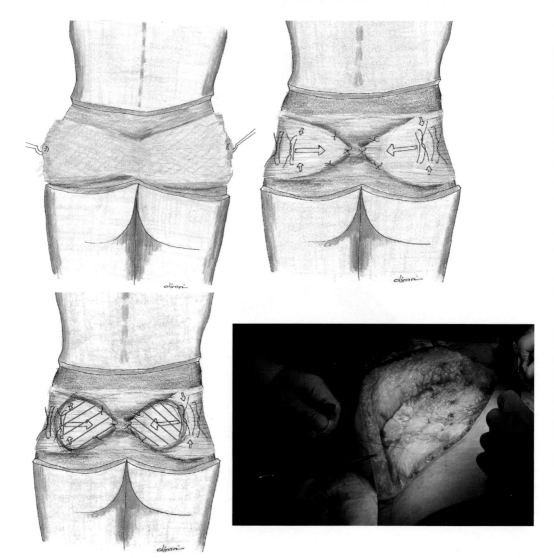

Fig. 6. Posterior view demonstration of the gluteal superficial fascial system ("gluteal SMAS") reconstruction, before mediovertical tightening (*top left*) and during the adipofascial shift (*top right*). Red cross-hatched area is the region of maximum projection immediately postoperatively (*bottom left*). Intraoperative view of the vertical tightening of the gluteal SFS (*bottom right*).

too far cranially owing to a lower incision line marked in the abdominal skin fold. Consequently, the mons pubis, which is often sagging and slackened, is not lifted. In more severe cases, the lower incision line can be extended caudally in a box-shaped manner into the mons pubis region, thus achieving a more effective tightening. Nevertheless, a distance of 6 to 7 cm to the upper vulva commissure should be respected (Fig. 11).

For the combination technique—particularly indicated in patients with massive weight loss (MWL)—the marking is initiated in accordance to the original technique for an inner thigh lift. Then the upper horizontal abdominal incision line of the modified technique is integrated and a large

abdominal resection area results, which emends an extensive abdominal as well as a lateral and inner thigh slackening (Fig. 12).

At the end of the patient's marking, important vector lines are marked to allow a medio-cranial rotation of the gluteal and thigh lift and a consecutive sculpturing of the waist (Fig. 13).

Operation techniques

General considerations

MWL patients may present with a difficult airway, thus an experienced anesthesia team should be employed. Hypothermia may occur in these operations because of the long operative times, which

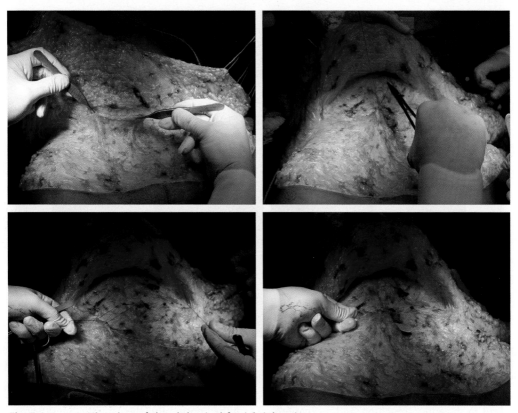

Fig. 7. Intraoperative view of the abdominal fascial tightening.

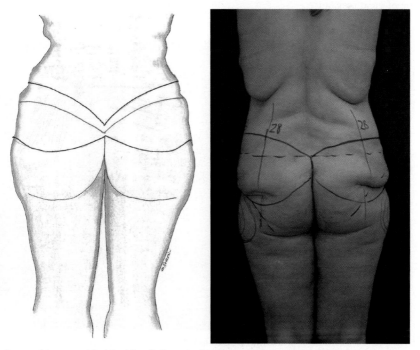

Fig. 8. Posterior markings are identical in all three techniques. Blue lines indicate the incision lines and red line indicates the resulting scar line (*left*). Preoperative markings, blue lines indicate the incision lines (*right*).

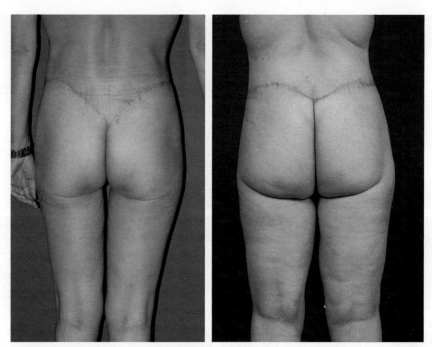

Fig. 9. Postoperative posterior view after a body lift procedure. Note the accentuation of the gluteal form by a sharp-angled scar course into the gluteal furrow (*left*). However, a higher and more straight horizontal scar course can result in a long and unesthetic gluteal furrow (*right*).

can lead to shivering, crouching, and an inappropriate cramping postoperatively—all leading to increased tension on the wounds. Preheated infusions, electrically heated blankets, and preheated beds can all be of great assistance.

When positioning the patient, it must be considered that large excesses of tissue can become compressed, a situation that can then lead to necroses and should be controlled by the surgeon. The entire team must bear these considerations in mind when

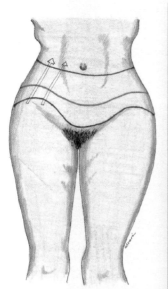
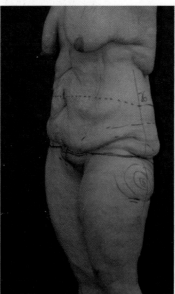
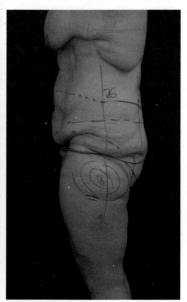

Fig. 10. Front view demonstration of the anterior markings in the modified technique. Blue lines indicate the incision course and red line indicates the resulting scar line. Arrows indicate the inward rotation of the anterolateral thigh flap (*left*). Preoperative markings, blue lines indicate the incision lines (*center and right*).

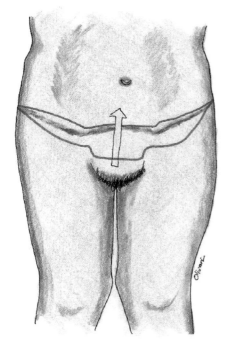

Fig. 11. Front view demonstration of the box-shaped markings in cases with moderate to severe mons pubis sagging, in primary and secondary procedures.

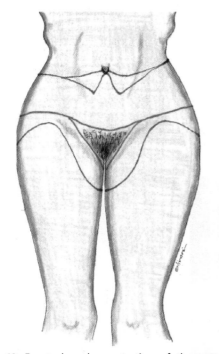

Fig. 12. Front view demonstration of the anterior markings in the combination technique. Blue lines indicate the incision course and red line indicates the resulting scar line.

positioning the patient. In a prone position in particular, pressure necroses can form around the periorbital regions and at the breasts [17].

Dorsal access

Ideally, the operation is performed by two surgeons, a medical assistant, and a surgery nurse so that parallel surgical operations can be performed on each side. After intubation and the insertion of a urinary bladder catheter, the patient is turned to the prone position and padded appropriately. Next, wide-area infiltration of tumescent solution (1 L of Ringer solution and one ampule of Suprarenin) is performed until satisfactory tissue turgor is achieved.

A skin incision is made along the superior mark and is taken down to the level of the underlying superficial fascia, which is exposed using the Harmonic ultrasound scalpel that separates the superficial lamellar fat from the subfascial lobular fat. Next, the dissection is performed inferiorly just above the robust white superficial fascia. This dissection just above the superficial fascia diverges considerably from the original technique by Lockwood, who resected below the fascia. The authors believe that leaving this fascia attached to the deep fat is similar to leaving the gluteal SMAS in place to be used in much the same manner as the SMAS is used in facelifts. The fascia is first pierced through shortly before reaching the inferior resection line so that, upon later skin closure, the SFS, which now adheres to the skin and no longer to the deep fat, can be reconstructed. The adhesions in the area of the lateral buttocks are released caudally until the gluteal fold before the dissection is continued to the lateral thigh below the superficial fascia. This allows dissection to be performed further on the aponeurosis of the tensor fascia lata muscle. The subsequent large-area mobilization of the lateral thigh skin is performed bluntly to few-fingers width to just above the knee through the use of the Lockwood dissector.

With this type of dissection, the waist and gluteal fat now hangs to the lateral side and is covered with a robust fascial structure. This is particularly suited for autologous buttock augmentations, as usually flattened buttocks are present. For this purpose, two to three 1/0 ethibond threads (Ethicon, Somerville, New Jersey) are sutured from the side to the middle through the fascia so that the fat on the side is displaced to the middle of the buttocks. For the cranial rotation and repositioning, three to four 1/0 Ethibond threads (Ethicon) are sutured from caudal to cranial through the more medial parts of the fascia. When tying the sutures, the vertical threads should cross the horizontal threads and cover them. As a result of this deep fascial firm lifting, the previously loosened skin–soft-tissue

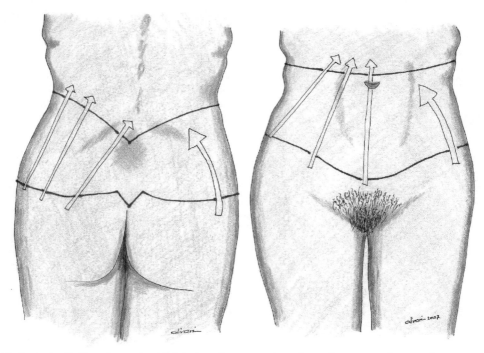

Fig. 13. Posterior (*left*) and anterior (*right*) view demonstration of rotation vectors for a waist accentuation. A barrel-shaped contour can be avoided in this way.

flap is translated well in the cranial direction in a way that reduces much of the tension on the subsequent skin closure. These maneuvers also lead to sculpting of the waist.

The extended mobilization and detachment of the adhesion zones allow an enormous tightening of the skin. The stretching and resection of the skin soft-tissue surplus should always be performed by a "leading" surgeon whose responsibility it is to ensure a symmetrical resection. To be able to reliably determine the extent of resection so that neither under- or overcorrection occurs, clamps should be used for temporary wound approximation. The marked vector lines (best tattooed using methylene blue) are incised, from medial to lateral, and adjusted for maximum tension. The resections may entail going past the original inferior marks. The medial, central, and lateral flaps arising in this way are measured precisely in the tensed condition for a symmetrical resection, which can now be performed between the clamps (Fig. 14).

The subsequent reconstruction of the SFS is performed using PDS 2×0 (Ethicon). The SFS is very stable, and when it is being pleated it is all the more important to grasp as little fat tissue as

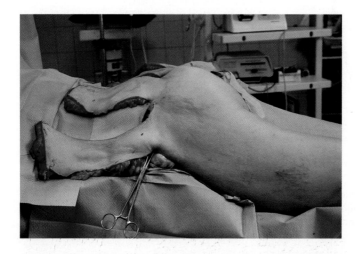

Fig. 14. Intraoperative demonstrating the prone position of the posterior medial, central, and lateral tissue flaps, which have to be excised between the clamps.

possible to avoid the development of fat necroses. After the repositioning and fixation of the SFS, the wound edges are further approximated, with the wound being closed in layers using resorbable suture material. Two drains are then placed in the back region and buried in the wound for turning. Before the patient is turned, a temporary closure of the lateral skin surplus dog-ear is performed using a stapler and an Opsite film. After turning the patient to a supine position, any required tightening of the abdomen and the thighs can now be performed, differentially depending on the specific indication.

Original technique

This technique is indicated with moderate lower abdominal slackening, severe upper abdominal slackening, and conditions after previously performed abdominoplasties. The incision course passes from the inner side of the thighs, runs steeply curved over the iliac crest, and then follows downward in the direction of the gluteal furrow. This method is particularly suitable when the main slackening occurs at the inner and outer sides of the thighs and the abdominal region is only moderately affected. A displacement and reinsertion of the umbilicus are not performed here, as the upper epigastrium is stretched not by lateral pulling (in contrast with the vertical pulling achieved in conventional abdominoplasties). This can be successfully repositioned by a combining incision at the height of the often sagging mons pubis. The guideline for measuring the extent of skin and soft-tissue tightening between the umbilicus to the symphysis is 60% hairless, 40% haired. The resultant scar has a "high-cut bikini" appearance and can be placed steep or shallow depending on the patient's wishes.

Modified technique

If the slackening of the abdominal skin is more severe, the use of the modified procedure is recommended [11]. This is performed essentially as a "high-lateral-tension abdominoplasty" with subsequent thigh and buttock lifting. The inferior incision is marked ventrally as it is with the conventional abdominoplasty; however, the lateral superior incision ends do not taper to a lateral point, but instead remain almost parallel to the inferior incision in the planed section to be resected.

Combination procedure

Many patients after MWL show a significant redundancy of skin and soft tissue in the body trunk and thigh areas. For this reason, the authors have endorsed a combination procedure since 1999 for severely slackened abdominal skin and inner thighs

that combines the benefits of the original and modified techniques. A combination of both procedures was an obvious thing to do: with the modified procedure, the slackened abdominal skin can be mobilized far cranially with a connecting incision above the pubic hairline. Although this maneuver requires a reinsertion of the umbilicus, it allows a further resection of soft tissue. Furthermore, if a rectus diastasis is present, a fascial doubling can be performed. This additionally allows an optimal stretching of the upper and lower abdomen on account of the high lateral incision course.

With conventional inner thigh lifts, only a purely vertical stretching could be reached by straight vertical pulling and fixation at the periosteum. Scar dehiscence and vulva distortion often resulted, which also entailed additional problems.

The combination technique enables an additional lateral rotation of the inner thigh skin to the vertical lifting. In this way, the strongest pulling is displaced cranially where the thigh skin can be fixated on the abdominal scarpa fascia. Moreover, an inner thigh wound can be placed free of tension and distortion in the groin so that it is exposed to only minimal vertical pulling.

With all techniques, the dissection level is performed above the scarpa fascia, entailing a number of key advantages: long-lasting swellings can be prevented because the underlying lymphatic vessels are preserved, and the stretching of the SFS craniomedially provides an additional "inner traction" on the deep-penetrating fascia system of the thigh. The SFS is then fixated with 1/0 Ethibond sutures (Ethicon) to the anterior rectus fascia. At a height of three-finger breadth below the umbilicus, the scarpa fascia is then pierced through and further dissection and mobilization of the abdominal flap are performed cranially on the anterior rectus fascia. The central supraumbilical adhesion zone is sharply dissected between both rectus muscles, preserving the laterally incoming perforator vessels.

In cases of rectus diastasis and/or abdominal fascial laxity, an anterior rectus fascia doubling is performed in one or several vertical or additionally transverse infraumbilical directions. Undermining may also have to be performed more laterally to prevent bulging in the midline. The umbilicus is now fixated at 3, 6, and 9 o'clock on the anterior rectus fascia, and resection of surplus tissue is performed in the usual manner. The new position of the umbilicus is marked, and a small, distally based triangular pedicular flap is incised, through which the umbilicus is pulled and sutured with a few Baroudi sutures in a tension-free manner. Before this, extensive periumbilical fat should be removed, continuing up cranially in the midline until a "Champagne groove" is created. After temporary wound closure with clamps, the SFS can now be re-constructed using PDS 2×0 (Ethicon). A multilayer wound closure with 3×0 and 4×0 monocryl (Ethicon) follows before intracuticular suturing is performed. Because of the wound length, 3×0 monocryl rapid (Ethicon) is recommended, thus making removal of the suture superfluous.

Postoperative care

Because of the extensive wound area, a single dose of antibiotics is administered. The patient is monitored 24 hours in the intensive or intermediate care unit. To ensure an optimal tissue turgor and appropriate microcirculation, 2500 mL of Ringer solution is provided over 24 hours. Furthermore, laboratory checks for electrolytes and hemoglobin are performed. The patient is placed in a beach-chair position on an alternating-pressure air mattress in an electronically adjustable bed. Thrombosis prophylaxis is administered using low-molecular heparins. The patient is given an individualized patient controlled analgesia (PCA) pump and is mobilized on the first day postoperatively. The average duration of hospitalization is 6 days. Before discharge, the patient should be fitted with a compression garment, which should be stringently worn for at least 6 to 8 weeks.

Result prognosis

A realistic prognosis for the outcome of the operation represents the basis on which the patient builds trust, the operation is planned, and the outcome of the operation is assessed. The translation test by Aly has proven itself to be worthwhile in clinical practice [18]. In this test the patient is asked to grasp his or her tissue surplus at the height of the waist and pull the excess tissue firmly upwards. The visible skin lift and body contour obtained in this way reliably forecasts the outcome of the thigh appearance after lower body lift operations. The best results can be achieved with a normal body mass index (BMI) of less than 25. If the BMI is too high, the patient must be informed that the result to be expected will be exponentially inferior. The upper limit for MWL surgery should not exceed a BMI of 32.

Problems and solutions

The authors evaluated their results retrospectively from the years 1995 to 2006 and collected data from more than 500 body lift operations. A list of the main problems and solutions encountered is shown in Box 2.

Operation time

Depending on patients' clinical findings, the authors' operations lasted initially from 6 to 9

Box 2:   Problems and solutions

- Operation time
- Symmetry
- Wound-healing disorders, perfusion disorders
- Scarring
- Seromas
- Buttock projection
- Waist formation
- Blood loss
- Infections
- Thrombosis

---

hours. As additional risks can arise from this long and strenuous operation time (eg, long periods of susceptibility to contamination, surgeons' fatigue, long anesthesia, drying out of the wounds), improvements to modify the procedure time were sought.

The authors eventually settled on performing the operation with only a single turn, starting in a prone position. This decreased operation time considerably, and it became possible for two teams to operate simultaneously. The optimal make-up consisted of two operation teams, each with two surgeons, one medical assistant, and an operating nurse. However, one surgeon should assume a lead role for the whole team, especially considering that equal resection needs to be achieved with a defined and symmetrical degree of stretching.

Symmetry

With the initial three-position/two-turn approach, asymmetric scar courses were noted, despite meticulous planning and an exact marking of the (standing) patient. This asymmetry was due to the lateral positioning not allowing for effective control of symmetry during the operation. The lateral positioning entailed that checking of a symmetric resection tension was not possible.

Lateral positioning can never be performed in a manner that exactly mirrors the positioning performed for the other side. Even minor changes in gluteal inclination lead to considerable distortions and, therefore, to inconsistent resection courses.

The positioning described above, on the other hand, proved to be of great use, as under the management of a single surgeon simultaneous and comparable resection and tension could be established. To ensure symmetry, it also proved useful to divide operation areas into precisely defined sectors using suitable vector lines (see Fig. 13).

Apart from a precise resection and preparation, precise intraoperative positioning is also important. Before prepping, the patient should be checked to make sure that he or she is lying straight and is not contorted.

Wound-healing disorders/perfusion disorders

Body lift operations are in principle large-flap operations. A precise knowledge of the vascular anatomy is necessary to prevent the operation from ending in a disaster.

Blood supply of the abdomen

Although in the past it was recommended that an extensive as possible undermining be performed to allow a tension-free wound closure, from today's perspective only the midline adhesion zones described by Lockwood should be released to provide the conditions for a tension-free wound closure. The supraumbilical undermining in the midline should only be a palm's width to preserve as many muscle perforators as possible. Nevertheless, the wound closure should still be performed in a tension-free manner to ensure as few problems as possible with respect to the flap perfusion [19].

Blood supply of the back

In the back, it is not advisable to undermine the superior midline flap tip that extends into the rima ani. Vessels in this region can be easily destroyed if the area is undermined; when combined with the compression from lying on this region postoperatively, necrosis can easily occur (Fig. 15).

Blood supply of the buttocks

In the distal part of the buttocks, the perforators from the two gluteal arteries are both powerful and dominant. This means that extensive undermining can indeed be performed, unless this affects the extended perianal region (see Fig. 15).

Blood supply of the thigh

Knowledge of the perfusion in the thigh area is of decisive importance for ensuring a complication-free outcome, as discontinuous undermining often has to be performed all the way caudally to the knee. One should consider that the dorsal part of the thigh, with its underlying small and delicate vessels, should not be damaged. The lateral aspect up to the front of the thigh can, however, be freed from the muscle layer without significant consequences. Here, it is important to dissect precisely on the tendon layer and not too superficially as otherwise the subcutaneous vascular plexus might be destroyed. During the authors' early experience with the use of lateral positioning, impairment of blood perfusion was observed within the lateral undermined skin owing to increased and prolonged local pressure.

Wound-healing problems represent the most frequent complication after such skin-lifting operations; they are the rule rather than the exception. Directly after the operation, erroneous repositioning or, indeed, excessive mobilization can lead to wound dehiscence. Here, ongoing training of the nursing staff and information for patients and their dependents can be helpful. A compression garment should be considered only with reservations. Although this might prevent seromas, it might compromise the microcirculation and wound healing at the incision line.

The authors employ a class 1 compression garment only after removal of the drains, whenever the patient is mobile. Secondary wound-healing disorders are usually observed if the suture material is perforated. Suture granulomas are common and lead to local infections with wound openings. In patients with gastric bypass in particular, important parameters must be monitored for wound healing: proteins, vitamin C, zinc, blood glucose, and hemoglobin levels. Later complications can usually be attributed to smaller or larger seromas.

Scarring

With major operations such as the body lift, large and long scars are created. In addition to the length and course of the scar, its width is also important

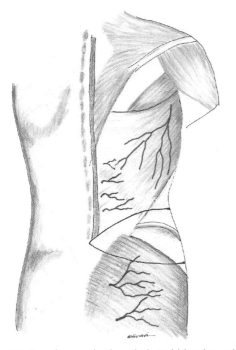

Fig. 15. Dorsal upper back and gluteal blood supply.

for the patient's ultimate assessment of the outcome.

Publications on the superficial connective tissue system by Lockwood in the early 1990s have brought along both a new understanding and respect to scar formation. As a result of the dissection on the level of the superficial tissue in the buttock area, a stable layer becomes available through which the deep-lying fat tissue of the buttocks can be rotated upwards with the strong fascial connective tissue layer. This consequently pulls the caudal skin flap upwards, a phenomenon that can improve the gluteal fold and/or cellulite.

The course of the scar is of similar importance. The surgeon has the option of individually shaping the scar course before and during the body lift procedure. The patient should be informed in detail about the consequences of the operation and any aesthetic problems that might arise.

Seroma

Because of the large area of the wounds, accumulations of wound fluid (seromas) can also present postoperative problems. At the lateral thigh in particular, seromas can occur in the knee region on account of gravity. Seroma formation cannot be prevented with any degree of certainty [5,10,14].

A diligent fitting of drains is absolutely necessary, although some authors disagree on this. Suction-assisted drains in the area of the lateral outer thigh until they reach less than 30 mL within 24 hours have proven to be useful here. The latter has far superior and more continuous aspiration properties than a regular aspiration drainage catheter.

Furthermore, the deep-fixation sutures as described by Baroudi are also helpful for achieving tissue contact and avoiding dead space that could preclude accumulations of fluid [20]. Over the last couple of years, the use of the ultrasonically activated Harmonic scalpel has demonstrated its potential for reducing seroma formation. Studies are being conducted to delineate the potential use of this instrument in the reduction of seromas in circumferential body lift procedures [21].

Buttock projection

In patients who experienced severe weight loss, it can frequently be observed that the buttocks become very flattened and ptotic owing to fat loss and tissue laxity. With previous surgical procedures and also body lifts, flat buttocks often occurred postoperatively.

Some surgeons prefer to use local subcutaneous flaps to increase buttocks projection. The authors prefer not to use flaps in this area as the resultant flaps may be injured from the pressure of sitting on them. The authors have opted for leaving behind as much buttocks tissue in its natural position as possible by performing the suprafascial resection described above. This "autologous tissue augmentation" is optimally perfused because undermining or displacement does not occur as it does with a flap mobilization. With this maneuver, a reconstruction of the deeper tissue is also possible, which tends to become lax in a manner different from the overlying skin. For this reason, it makes sense to allow a multilayer reconstruction and to consider the various reconstruction vectors. Comparable to facelift operations, a bi-vectoral remodeling can be performed in this region (Fig. 16).

Waist formation

When body lift surgery was first established, waist formation was insufficiently addressed. Frequently, barrel-shaped trunks were observed because the upper skin soft-tissue flap did not match the lower soft-tissue flap in diameter. Often in earlier body lifts, the sagging tissue was simply pulled up like a pair of trousers. Several tricks were therefore developed to provide the basis for sculpturing an aesthetically pleasant waist contour.

It is important to note that after waist contouring, the extent of the lower tissue after dissection in the back area is greater than that of the upper tissue. Consequently, a wound closure has to be managed by tissue crimping for optimal adaptation.

Upon wound closure—especially in the lateral aspect of the body lift—it must be ensured that all tissue layers are reconstructed separately and that they allow a certain degree of reattachment in the area of the waist. Otherwise, an empty cavity and a feared tent shape results.

If a complete abdominoplasty is performed in the context of a modified body lift, an external muscle belt can be applied to improve the accentuation of the waist. This involves excision, overcrossing, and non-resorbable suturing of two U-shaped fascial tissue strips in the region of the anterior rectus fascia above the umbilicus. In this way, achieving an extreme accentuation of the waist above the umbilicus can be attempted, which leads to the formation of an attractive body contour (Fig. 17).

Infection

The fear of an infection spreading rapidly after body lifts is justified but fortunately extremely rare. The large wound cavities and the raised adhesion zones that prevent any transgression to neighboring section allow microorganisms to spread freely in a large operative wound. Ameliorating surgical maneuvers that should be considered include (1) operating swiftly, (2) operating carefully, (3)

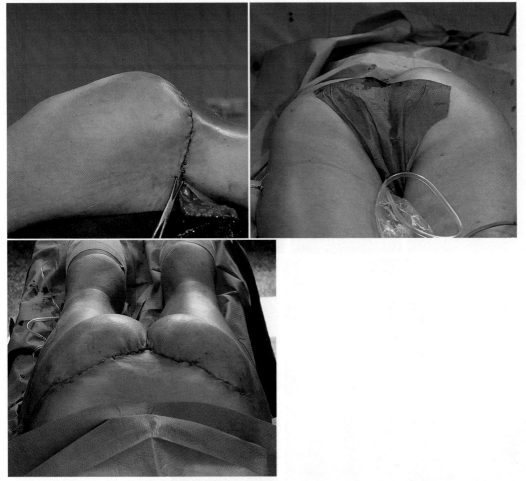

Fig. 16. Satisfactory intraoperative upper gluteal projection after repositioning by autologous fat augmentation on the patient's right side in lateral view (*top left*), inferior view (*top right*), and bilaterally in superior view (*bottom*).

avoiding tissue drenching, and (4) providing a perioperative antibiotic-prophylaxis. In individual cases with risk factors for infections (higher BMI, smokers, recent operations in wound area, etc), a postoperative antibiotic treatment is also recommended.

By using these precautions, the authors have observed over the course of the years only three

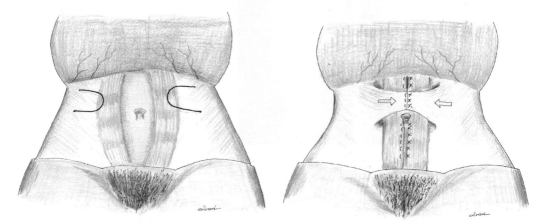

Fig. 17. Formation and tightening of an external muscle belt.

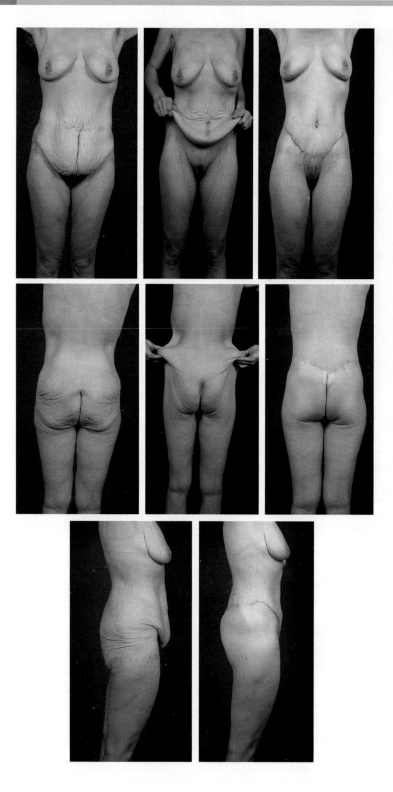

Fig. 18. Front (*top*), posterior (*middle*), and lateral (*bottom*) view of a 37-year-old patient after a weight reduction of 62 kg preoperatively (*left*), active demonstration of the excess tissue and the achievable improvements (translation test) (*center*), and 6 weeks postoperatively (*right*) after circumferential suprafascial dermatolipectomy.

infections—rapidly spreading abdominal wall phlegmons. The immediate surgical wound treatment as well as the fitting of a suction-lavage drain produced good results.

Blood loss

Most patients after gastric bypass suffer from anemia. This must be recognized and treated accordingly before the patient is operated on. The large

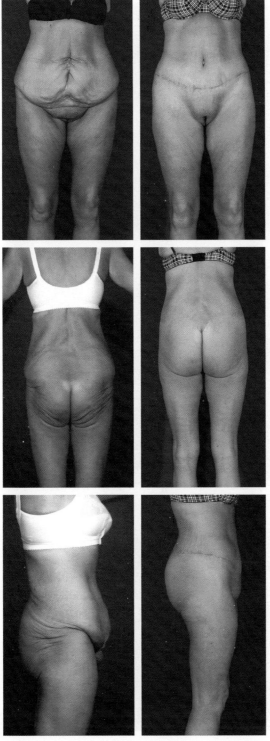

Fig. 19. Front (*top*), posterior (*middle*), and lateral (*bottom*) view of a 42-year-old patient after a weight reduction of 70 kg preoperatively (*left*) and 8 weeks postoperatively (*right*) after circumferential suprafascial dermatolipectomy.

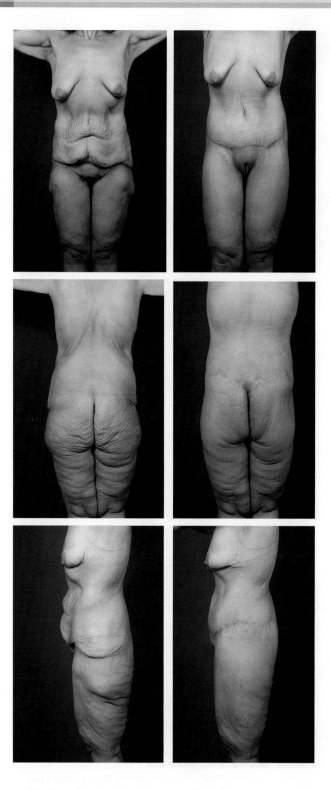

Fig. 20. Front (*top*), posterior (*middle*), and lateral (*bottom*) view of a 46-year-old patient after a weight reduction of 102 kg preoperatively (*left*) and 12 weeks postoperatively (*right*) after circumferential suprafascial dermatolipectomy.

and well-perfused wound area, as well as the partly indirect dissection using the Lockwood canula, can already lead to greater blood loss. Even if symptoms of anemia do not occur directly during the operation, they can nevertheless occur secondarily owing to the large wound area, even if hemostasis was performed meticulously. Consequently, patients have to be informed preoperatively about the possibility of treatment by blood transfusion. Autohemotherapy can be considered, but is usually refused by most experienced clinicians. For legal reasons, however, the patient must be informed about this option. A patient who does not agree to consent to a possible blood transfusion should be excused from treatment Fig. 18.

Thrombosis

Because of the extended operation time and the size of the wound area (and the potential fat trauma this entails), the risk of thrombosis also increases. The patient should be asked about his or her medical history regarding thrombosis and personal habits such as smoking; in all cases, appropriate prophylaxis should be considered.

As a standard procedure in the Department of Plastic and Reconstructive Surgery, thrombosis prophylaxis is performed using low–molecular-weight heparin in a weight-adapted manner. Also, the support of intraoperative compression treatment of the lower legs by bandaging with sterile elastic is standardized. Furthermore, a postoperative beach-chair positioning and early mobilization are mandatory in the authors' patients' antithrombosis arrangements. In the United States, intermittent compression pumps are considered standard care and can be considered an alternative to compression stockings.

The authors also administer circulation-promoting measures such as infusions within the first 3 days, whereby the patients receive 2 to 3 L of Ringer-lactate for dilution of the circulating blood. To date, the authors have observed three deep–leg-vein thromboses as well as a single pulmonary embolism event in their patient collective without a single fatality Figs. 19 and 20.

References

[1] Anderson WA, Greene GW, Forse RA, et al. Weight loss and health outcomes in African Americans and whites after gastric bypass surgery. Obesity 2007;15(6):1455–63.

[2] Buchwald H, Williams SE. Bariatric surgery worldwide 2003. Obes Surg 2004;14(9): 1157–64.

[3] Richter DF, Stoff A, Uckunkaya E, et al. Perils and pitfalls in lower body lifts. Int J Adi Tissue 2007; 1:12–23.

[4] Gonzales-Ulloa M. Belt lipectomy. Br J Plast Surg 1961;13:179–86.

[5] Aly AS, Cram AE, Chao M, et al. Belt lipectomy for circumferential truncal excess: the University of Iowa experience. Plast Reconstr Surg 2003; 111(1):398–413.

[6] Lockwood TE. Superficial fascial system (SFS) of the trunk and extremities: a new concept. Plast Reconstr Surg 1991;87(6):1009–18.

[7] Lockwood TE. Transverse flank-thigh-buttock lift with superficial fascial suspension. Plast Reconstr Surg 1991;87(6):1019–27.

[8] Lockwood TE. Lower body lift with superficial fascial system suspension. Plast Reconstr Surg 1993;92(6):1112–22.

[9] Hurwitz DJ. Single-staged total body lift after massive weight loss. Ann Plast Surg 2004;52(5): 435–41 [discussion: 441].

[10] Kenkel JM. Body contouring surgery after massive weight loss. Plast Reconstr Surg 2006; 117(1):33–45.

[11] Lockwood TE. The role of excisional lifting in body contour surgery. Clin Plast Surg 1996; 23(4):695–712.

[12] Lockwood TE. Maximizing aesthetics in lateral-tension abdominoplasty and body lifts. Clin Plast Surg 2004;31(4):523–37.

[13] Nemerofsky RB, Oliak DA, Capella JF. Body lift: an account of 200 consecutive cases in the massive weight loss patient. Plast Reconstr Surg 2006;117(2):414–30.

[14] Rohrich RJ, Gosman AA, Conrad MH, et al. Simplifying circumferential body contouring: the central body lift evolution. Plast Reconstr Surg 2006;118(2):525–35 [discussion: 536–8].

[15] Strauch B, Herman C, Rohde C, et al. Perils and pitfalls in lower body lifts: mid-body contouring in the post-bariatric surgery patient. Plast Reconstr Surg 2006;117(7):2200–11.

[16] Reichenberger MA, Stoff A, Richter DF. Body contouring surgery in the massive weight loss patient. Chirurg 2007;78(4):326–34 [in German].

[17] Rubin JP, Nguyen V, Schwentker A. Perioperative management of the post-gastric-bypass patient presenting for body contour surgery. Clin Plast Surg 2004;31(4):601–10.

[18] Aly AS. Body contouring after massive weight loss. St. Louis (MO): Quality Medical Publishing; 2006.

[19] Huger WE Jr. The anatomic rationale for abdominal lipectomy. Am Surg 1979;45(9):612–7.

[20] Baroudi R, Moraes M. Philosophy, technical principles, selection, and indications in body contouring surgery. Aesthetic Plast Surg 1991; 15:1–18.

[21] Stoff A, Reichenberger MA, Richter DF. Comparing the ultrasonically-activated scapel (Harmonic™) versus high-frequency electrocautery on postoperative serous drainage in massive-weight-loss surgery. Plast Reconstr Surg 2007; 120:1092–3.

ELSEVIER
SAUNDERS

CLINICS IN
PLASTIC
SURGERY

Clin Plastic Surg 35 (2008) 73–91

Gluteal Contouring Surgery in the Massive Weight Loss Patient

Robert F. Centeno, MD, MBA[a],*, Constantino G. Mendieta, MD, FACS[b],
V. Leroy Young, MD, FACS[a]

- Platypygia in the patient who has lost a massive amount of weight
- Topical anatomic landmarks
- Clinical anatomy
- Classification system
  - *Task 1: Evaluate the frame*
  - *Task 2: Evaluate the gluteus maximus muscle*
  - *Task 3: Evaluate the four junction points of the muscle and the frame*
  - *Task 4: Evaluate degree of ptosis from lateral view*
- Autologous gluteal augmentation with flaps

- *Autologous flap indications*
- *Complications*
- Autologous fat transfer
- Adjunctive excisional techniques for gluteal enhancement
- Alloplastic implant augmentation techniques
  - *Submuscular*
  - *Intramuscular*
  - *Subfascial*
- Technique selection and decision algorithm
- Summary
- References

A growing demand for gluteal augmentation in the United States has been attributed to multiple factors, such as changing demographics, improving body-contouring techniques, and evolving esthetic preferences. The population that has sustained massive weight loss (MWL), with its severe deformities in the buttocks region, is no exception to this trend. This article describes anatomic issues, a system for esthetic evaluation, surgical techniques, and an algorithm to assist with decision making for gluteal contouring in patients who have lost a massive amount of weight. The results obtained with autologous tissue in combination with the circumferential body lift (CBL) cannot match those typical of gluteal augmentation in patients who have not lost significant weight and have little skin excess. Nevertheless, the

gluteal esthetics of patients who have sustained MWL can be enhanced greatly with an autologous tissue flap at the time of CBL. Furthermore, a subset of MWL patients can benefit from autologous fat transfer as the primary or an adjunctive mode of gluteal contouring. Adjunctive excisional techniques, such as a posterior thigh lift or an infragluteal "diamond" lift, can refine results. Alloplastic implants remain a less frequently used option in the population that has experienced MWL.

Platypygia in the patient who has lost a massive amount of weight

Anatomic changes that occur in the gluteal region contribute to platypygia (flattening of the

[a] BodyAesthetic Plastic Surgery & Skincare Center, 969 North Mason Road, Suite 170, St. Louis, MO 63141, USA
[b] 2310 South Dixie Highway, Coconut Grove, FL 33133, USA
* Corresponding author.
E-mail address: rfcentenomd@bodyaesthetic.com (R.F. Centeno).

doi:10.1016/j.cps.2007.08.009

buttocks) as we age. Several changes may coexist, including accumulation of subcutaneous adipose tissue around the gluteal region, loss of adipose volume in the buttock, postmenopausal accumulation of intra-abdominal fat coupled with rectus diastasis, skin laxity and buttock ptosis, increased hip width, and lengthening of the infragluteal fold [1–3]. All of these natural changes contribute to decreased buttock projection and ptosis, and any one of them may prompt patients to seek contouring of the gluteal region. Additionally, dramatic weight loss may cause significant adipose tissue loss in the buttock that exacerbates the skin laxity and platypygia seen with normal aging. The CBL effectively addresses many of these concerns; unfortunately, however, the buttocks tend to appear even more flattened if aggressive lifting is performed to improve contour of the thighs and lower back. Any preexisting platypygia that is worsened by a CBL may erode patient satisfaction among those who have experienced MWL (Fig. 1).

Patients who have lost a large amount of weight are affected greatly by platypygia, in part because their weight loss—whether through diet or surgery—often occurs in an uneven manner. Data suggest that adipose tissues in certain body regions are more resistant to weight loss than are others [4]. The genetic programming of the resistant adipocytes differs from more responsive areas, which may mean that genetics influence different somatotypes, or body types. Following weight loss, the "apple" somatotype seems to have less adipose tissue in the gluteal region, whereas the "pear" tends to retain more tissue in this area. Regardless of body type, many MWL patients tend to lose gluteal volume and want to have this deformity addressed.

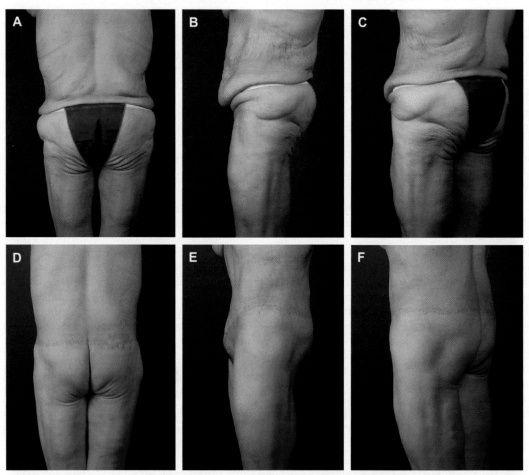

Fig. 1. Gluteal flattening effect of a CBL. (*A–C*) This 46-year-old woman had typical deformities following MWL, including platypygia. (*D–F*) Postoperative views demonstrate how a CBL can exacerbate platypygia. In addition, the straight incision makes her buttocks appear masculine, shorter, and more square after her CBL. (*From* Centeno RF. Autologous gluteal augmentation with circumferential body lift in the massive weight loss and aesthetic patient. Clin Plast Surg 2006;33:480; with permission.)

MWL patients also develop skeletal changes that may contribute to platypygia (Fig. 2). Morbid obesity equates to restrictive lung disease that has an obstructive component. Expiratory flow limitation in the supine position may lead to pulmonary hyperinflation and intrinsic positive end-expiratory pressure. This is believed to play a role in the positional orthopnea reported by obese patients [5,6]. Over time, the thoracic skeleton expands in obese patients to accommodate the increased need for functional reserve capacity and to accommodate hyperinflation. Thoracic kyphosis secondary to thoracic spine compression and anterior inclination of the pelvis also occur [7]. Inadequately treated postgastric bypass hypocalcemia and vitamin D malabsorption, secondary hypoparathyroidism, and independent negative bone remodeling modulated by sex hormone alterations or serum telopeptides also may worsen the weight-related skeletal alterations [8]. These changes seem to be permanent and tend to exacerbate any preexisting primary or secondary platypygia caused by loss of adipose tissue in the gluteal region after MWL.

Topical anatomic landmarks

Fig. 3 illustrates several superficial anatomic landmarks that have clinical relevance to gluteal augmentation with alloplastic implants or autologous tissue [9–16]. These landmarks provide a "road map" for surgical procedures and have significant implications for the postoperative appearance of specific gluteal features that are judged to be appealing by our society, including the sacral triangle, sacral dimples, and trochanteric depressions [17–19].

The iliac crest, which forms the superior border of the buttocks, is a palpable and often visible landmark for guiding incision placement in a buttock lift or the posterior portion of a CBL with autologous gluteal augmentation. To achieve a more esthetically pleasing postoperative result, the incision placement may vary superiorly or inferiorly with respect to the iliac crest. Advantages and disadvantages of higher and lower incision placement are presented in Box 1, but choosing an incision location requires a trade-off between waist definition and buttock elongation. In patients who have experienced MWL with a long history of obesity, good waist definition is nearly impossible to achieve regardless of where a CBL incision is placed, because many years of an expanded rib cage have left them with a "barrel chest" deformity (see Fig. 2) that cannot be corrected.

The posterior superior iliac spines (PSIS) form two distinct depressions called the sacral dimples that result from the confluence of the PSIS, the multifidus muscles, the lumbosacral aponeurosis, and the insertion of the gluteus maximus. These

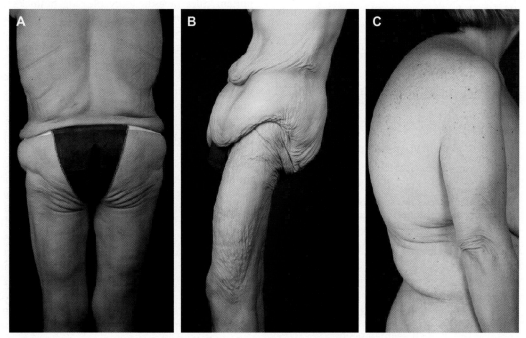

Fig. 2. Skeletal deformities encountered in patients who have experienced MWL include (*A*) a "barrel chest" from long-term expansion of the rib cage, (*B*) rotation of the pelvis, and (*C*) kyphosis. (*From* Centeno RF. Autologous gluteal augmentation with circumferential body lift in the massive weight loss and aesthetic patient. Clin Plast Surg 2006;33:481; with permission.)

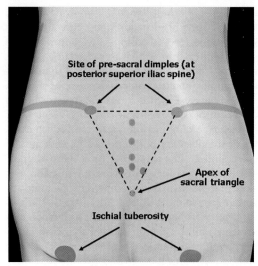

Site of pre-sacral dimples (at posterior superior iliac spine)

Apex of sacral triangle

Ischial tuberosity

Fig. 3. Superficial anatomic landmarks: iliac crest, posterior-superior iliac spine, sacral triangle, and ischial tuberosity. (*From* Centeno RF, Young VL. Clinical anatomy in aesthetic gluteal body contouring surgery. Clin Plast Surg 2006;33:348; with permission.)

anatomic depressions, which are characteristic of attractive buttocks, should be part of the buttock evaluation, and attempts can be made to create, define, or unmask this anatomic feature to improve surgical outcomes [17]. The sacral dimples also are good reference points for esthetic analysis and deformity classifications.

The sacral dimples serve as the superior corners of the "sacral triangle," which is defined by the two PSIS with the coccyx as the inferior border of the triangle [9,18]. Because it is esthetically

---

Box 1: Incision placement trade-offs

High incision
Advantages

Better maintains waist-to-hip ratio laterally

Disadvantages

Elongates buttocks
Limits flap placement so maximum
 projection is higher than ideal
Violates sacral triangle esthetic unit
Scar visible in some clothes

Low incision
Advantages

Shortens buttocks
Allows lower flap placement
Maintains sacral triangle aesthetic unit
Scar is well hidden, even in bikini

Disadvantages

Diminishes waist definition

---

pleasing, this triangle and its borders should be enhanced during surgery if possible. Liposuction or an "inverted dart" modification of the posterior CBL incision (Fig. 4) is useful for enhancing the sacral triangle [20,21]. A recent report on gluteal esthetic units (Fig. 5) explains how to enhance the sacral triangle and other gluteal units during body-contouring procedures [20]. The location of the sacral triangle feature should be marked and respected during augmentation with a tissue flap, transferred fat, or implants.

Another important topical landmark is the lateral trochanteric depression formed by the greater trochanter and insertions of thigh and buttocks muscles, including the gluteus medius, vastus lateralis, quadratus femoris, and gluteus maximus. This depression is important in the esthetics of an athletically toned buttock, although some ethnic groups (eg, African Americans and Hispanics in the United States) prefer that the trochanteric depressions not be emphasized or even filled if pronounced [19]. This anatomic landmark is useful when classifying buttock shape as round, square, A-shape, or V-shape (Fig. 6).

The infragluteal fold, which serves as the inferior border of the buttock proper, is formed by thick fascial insertions from the femur and pelvis through the intermuscular fascia to the skin. These structures create the fixed, well-defined subgluteal sulcus [2]. The infragluteal fold length and definition play important roles in esthetically pleasing buttocks. A longer infragluteal fold suggests an aged, ptotic, and deflated-looking buttock with skin and fascial excess. In contrast, a shorter infragluteal fold contributes to a full, taut, and youthful-looking buttock [1]. The ischial tuberosities, although not a part of the buttock proper, are the bony prominences upon which people sit.

Clinical anatomy

The integrity of superficial anatomic structures of the lateral trunk, posterior trunk, and gluteal region are most at risk for injury during the posterior portion of a CBL or buttock-flank lift. The iliohypogastric and ilioinguinal nerves are branches of the L1 nerve root. Originating in the sacral plexus, these nerves travel inferomedially between the transversus abdominis and internal oblique muscles. The iliohypogastric nerve divides into lateral and anterior cutaneous branches to supply the skin above the pubis and overlying the lateral gluteal region. CBL incisions made at or below the inguinal crease can put these nerves at risk.

The lateral cutaneous branches of the iliohypogastric and the intercostal nerves also can be entrapped laterally during a CBL. This might occur if

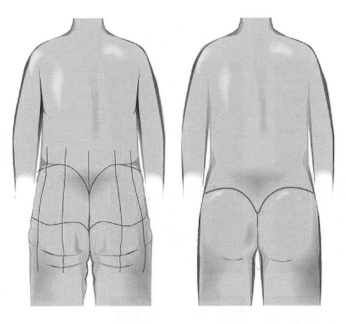

Fig. 4. Preoperative markings and postoperative position of the "inverted dart" modification to the posterior CBL incision. The patient in *Fig.* 1 would have benefited from this posterior incision, which we developed after she had surgery. (*From* Centeno RF, Young VL. Clinical anatomy in aesthetic gluteal body contouring surgery. Clin Plast Surg 2006;33:348; with permission.)

aggressive lateral plication of the external oblique muscle is performed to enhance waist definition or if "three-point" or quilting sutures are used laterally to close "dead space." Sensation to the gluteal region and lateral trunk has several sources: the dorsal rami of sacral nerve roots 3 and 4, the cutaneous branches of the iliohypogastric nerve arising from the L1 root, and the superior cluneal nerves originating from the L1, L2, and L3 roots and then passing over the iliac crest. The protective cutaneous sensation transmitted by these nerves is disrupted temporarily during a CBL, with or without auto-

augmentation. Therefore, patients must be counseled about the need for frequent positional changes and avoidance of heating pads to prevent pressure necrosis or burns. The long-term implications of dissecting these nerves during a CBL or autologous gluteal augmentation (AGA) have not been studied systematically.

Perfusion to the skin overlying the gluteal region is supplied by perforating branches of the superior and inferior gluteal arteries, both of which branch from the internal iliac artery. The lumbosacral region also is supplied by lumbar perforators. Some

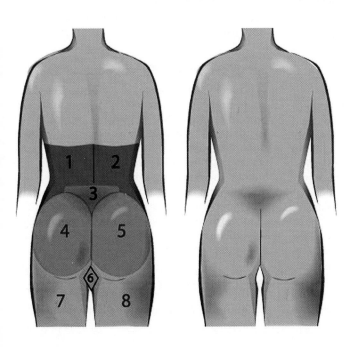

Fig. 5. The eight gluteal esthetic units: two symmetric flank units (1 and 2); sacral triangle unit (3); two symmetric buttock units (4 and 5); infragluteal "diamond" unit (6); and two symmetric thigh units (7 and 8). (*From* Centeno RF, Young VL. Clinical anatomy in aesthetic gluteal body contouring surgery. Clin Plast Surg 2006;33:349; with permission.)

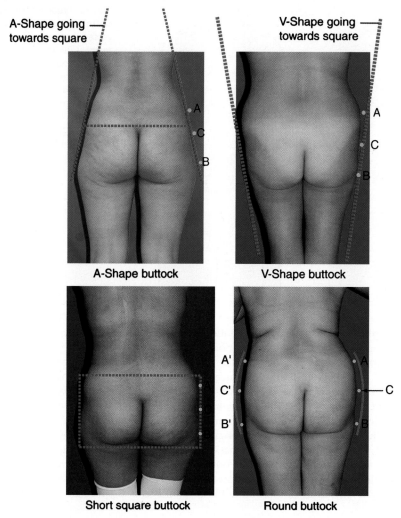

A-Shape going towards square

V-Shape going towards square

A-Shape buttock

V-Shape buttock

Short square buttock

Round buttock

Fig. 6. The four different buttock shapes: A-shape, V-shape, square, and round (*From* Mendieta CG. Classification system for gluteal evaluation. Clin Plast Surg 2006;33:335; with permission.)

of these perforators must be sacrificed during the posterior portion of a CBL, an AGA with CBL, or a buttock-flankplasty; however, the abundant vascular supply of the gluteal region provides robust perfusion to surrounding tissue flaps [22–24].

The fascial anatomy of the gluteal region greatly affects the esthetics of the aging buttock. In addition to volume loss and skin laxity, relaxation of the fascial "apron" contributes to gluteal ptosis. This superficial fascial "apron" is analogous to the superficial fascial system (SFS); its resection and tightening improve gluteal ptosis and play a significant role in the CBL procedure and AGA with CBL. Similar to the role played by the deep gluteal fascia as a strong retaining fascia in the subfascial approach to augmentation with implants, it also serves as a fixation point in AGA with CBL. The superficial apron and deep gluteal fascia fuse and become tightly adherent to form the infragluteal fold [2].

Classification system

To achieve the best esthetic shape, buttock contouring and gluteal augmentation need to be addressed concomitantly because they are interrelated. When approaching any patient who is interested in gluteal contouring, one should think in terms of contour first and augmentation second. For simplicity, the buttock should be thought of as containing two separate removable structures: the frame and the detachable gluteal muscle. Thorough gluteal evaluation entails four tasks that can be summarized only briefly here [25].

Task 1: Evaluate the frame

1. Determine if the pelvis is tall, intermediate, or short.

2. Determine the frame type (round, square, A- or V-shape) to help evaluate where liposuction may be indicated (see Fig. 6).
3. Evaluate point C (Fig. 7) and determine the degree of depression (none, mild, moderate, and severe) to decide if fat transfers are warranted. Also, assess whether any skin wrinkling is present at points A, B, or C.
4. Identify the sacral height, which should be less than one third of the intergluteal crease length. If the sacral length is equal to or greater than the crease length, the intergluteal crease may need to be lengthened visually by adding volume to the upper inner buttock or defining the sacral triangle area with liposuction. The inverted dart modification of the posterior CBL incision may be used to shorten a long intergluteal crease and restore proper proportions.

Task 2: Evaluate the gluteus maximus muscle

1. Determine if the patient has a tall, intermediate, or short gluteal muscle compared with its width. If the muscle is tall (2:1 ratio), use an anatomic implant or the moustache AGA flap (described below). If the muscle is short (1:1 ratio), use a round implant or the island AGA flap. Most patients fall in between (1–2:1 ratio), in which case a second criterion is needed. From the lateral view, identify where most of the gluteal volume lies (upper, middle, or lower part of the buttock). If most of the volume is in the upper buttock, an anatomic implant or moustache flap is best. If most of the volume is central, either flap or any implant could be used. If most of the volume is in the lower zone, a round implant or island flap should be used.
2. Identify whether the inferior gluteal base width is narrow, normal, or wide.

3. Evaluate all four quadrants of the muscle as sufficient or deficient (upper inner, upper outer, lower inner, and lower outer quadrants) to help determine where volume is needed.

Task 3: Evaluate the four junction points of the muscle and the frame

1. The upper inner gluteal/sacral junction usually requires some definition to look esthetic. If the area is flat and blunt, there may be excess fat in the sacral triangle, in which case liposuction is the best option. If there is a lack of volume at this junction, a flap or fat transfer may be necessary.
2. The intergluteal crease/leg junction also may require definition to achieve the infragluteal "diamond" esthetic unit, which should have a downward-sloping 45° angle between the lower margin of the intergluteal crease and the top of the inner thigh. If too much fullness exists, the inner infragluteal fold will appear as a horizontal line or an upward-sloping angle. If excess skin or tissue exists, consider liposuction or an infragluteal fold excision to recontour the "diamond" unit. This is common in ptotic buttocks often seen in MWL patients.
3. Evaluate the lower lateral gluteal/leg junction and the lateral midgluteal/hip junction. These areas should make a smooth transition. If there is a moderate or sharp demarcation point, consider fat transfers.

Task 4: Evaluate degree of ptosis from lateral view

1. Determine whether the patient has grade I, II, or III ptosis, which depends on the degree to which skin droops over the infragluteal fold. Grade III is characterized by a marked skin fold that may

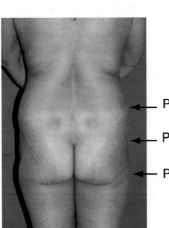

Point A, Upper lateral hip area

Point C, Mid-buttock area

Point B, Lateral leg area

Fig. 7. Consider points A, B, and C to help identify frame type. (*From* Mendieta CG. Classification system for gluteal evaluation. Clin Plast Surg 2006;33:334; with permission.)

extend onto the lateral thigh. The existence of skin laxity or wrinkling at points A, B, or C helps to identify whether ptosis is present. The patient may need AGA or an upper buttock lift (for grades II or III) or an infragluteal fold excision later (for grade III).

2. No ptosis is present if no skin droops below the infragluteal fold and the buttock volume is above the fold. A lack of ptosis does not mean that volume augmentation is not necessary. The lateral view also helps to determine if liposuction of the lumbosacral area is indicated to achieve improved gluteal contour.

Autologous gluteal augmentation with flaps

De-epithelialized flaps have been used in gluteal contouring during the last 3 decades [26–28]. Reports on the use of autologous tissue in preventing gluteal deformities with CBL also have been published, although they lacked significant detail and did not substantiate their potential for augmentation [15,16]; however, descriptions of the superior gluteal artery, inferior gluteal artery, and transverse lumbosacral back flaps and their vascular supplies have substantiated the clinical viability of using autologous tissue flaps for enhancing gluteal volume [23].

The natural evolution of what was learned in the literature review, combined with experience in alloplastic augmentation, led to the concept of using available, well-vascularized autologous tissue in the buttock region to address the gluteal deformities of MWL patients and the flattening effects of a CBL. Instead of discarding all tissue removed during the posterior portion of a CBL, it can be molded into the shape of an implant and inset beneath the CBL skin flaps. Various autologous flap designs emerged over time.

The first flap design, called an island AGA flap, simulates the round, nonanatomic design of submuscular gluteal implants (Fig. 8). This flap produces reasonable results, but long-term augmentation is modest with the island flap. Although its point of maximum projection is higher than ideal, it remains a viable option in the male patient who has experienced MWL and has a short, anthropometric pelvis and in those with preexisting lower pole fullness (Fig. 9).

Esthetic results achieved with island flaps are less than optimal, and the amount of volume that they produce is insufficient to overcome the gluteal flatness produced by a CBL in most MWL patients; however, experience gained with early flap designs led to the development of the moustache AGA flap (Fig. 10). The technical procedure for designing and insetting this flap has been described elsewhere

[20,29,30]. The moustache flap uses lower back and lateral flank tissue as a partial island and partial transposition flap based on perforators from the superior gluteal artery and lumbar perforators [24]. The anatomy of these perforators—as it relates to the moustache flap design—recently was documented in the literature as consistently being approximately 9 cm from the midline [31].

Inferomedial transposition of the "handlebar" portions of the moustache flap allows recruitment of additional tissue for augmentation purposes and lowers the point of maximum gluteal projection to the level of the mons pubis, which is considered the esthetic ideal. In addition, imbrication of the flap with sutures permits formation of a more anatomically shaped tissue mound that is reminiscent of anatomic gluteal implants. Because resection of tissue from the central area of the flap to allow easier insetting likely would decrease projection, the tissue volume in this area is included in the flap. The moustache flap is our preferred choice when significant, long-lasting esthetic augmentation is desired in patients who have experienced MWL (Figs. 11–13).

Autologous flap indications

Once AGA with CBL is chosen, the most appropriate flap design must be selected. The island flap produces the smallest volume of tissue and, consequently, the least amount of augmentation; however, it is indicated for minimizing the gluteal flattening effects of a CBL in patients who have sufficient preoperative buttock projection or do not desire increased gluteal volume. This flap should be used only for patients with adequate tissue overlying the sacrum. Inadequate postsacral tissue, which is typical among patients who have experienced MWL, often elicits complaints of pain in the coccyx or sacral area when sitting, and an island flap cannot produce needed padding over the sacrum. The island flap's point of maximum projection, which usually lies slightly above the transposed level of the mons pubis, is a location often preferred by men and by African American and Asian women, however [19].

The moustache flap is the design of choice when definitive augmentation is desired, especially for female patients who have experienced MWL. It yields the greatest amount of volume, produces superior esthetic results, and the augmentation achieved seems to be long lasting, at least during the 3 years of our experience. The flap is flexible in that its height and width can be adjusted to produce the amount of volume desired by the patient. A moustache flap potentially addresses the symptoms of postsacral tissue deficiency by maintaining a central bridge of tissue, which also maintains appropriate

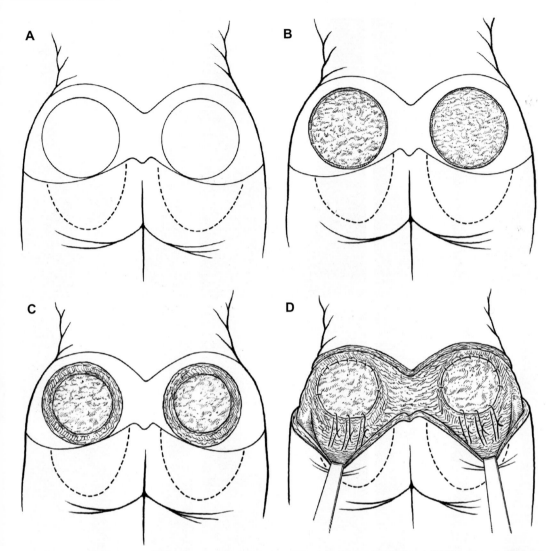

Fig. 8. Island AGA flap design. (*A, B*) The island flap is outlined and de-epithelialized. (*C*) The flap dissection is beveled down through the SFS and lumbosacral gluteal fascia, and surrounding excess tissue is removed down to the level of the lumbosacral fascia. This creates the two dermal "islands" of tissue. (*D*) The superior half of each island is imbricated (dermis to SFS), and the islands are anchored to the gluteal fascia at the desired level. As the inferior CBL skin flap is elevated and advanced over the AGA flap, the overlying CBL and underlying AGA flaps are attached together with #1 Vicryl Plus quilting sutures to reduce dead space. (*From* Centeno RF. Autologous gluteal augmentation with circumferential body lift in the massive weight loss and aesthetic patient. Clin Plast Surg 2006;33:482; with permission.)

flap position and reduces the risk for delayed wound healing in the central region of the posterior CBL incision. Because it recruits lateral trunk tissue inferomedially, the final point of transposed maximum projection is at the level of the mons pubis, which is the most generally accepted gluteal ideal. Patients with a body mass index (BMI) of less than 25 kg/m^2, skin laxity, buttocks ptosis, and platypygia after MWL are ideal candidates for a moustache flap.

Regardless of the flap design chosen, the volume of the flaps described can be adjusted as required by the clinical situation and the patient's wishes. Although larger flaps produce more augmentation, smaller ones are sometimes desired, especially if it becomes apparent that an increased margin of safety is needed to guarantee tissue perfusion or if a larger flap places excessive tension on the posterior CBL flaps. The only limitation to larger flap volume is the upper border of the skin-marking pattern used for a CBL. All autologous flaps can be "down-staged" intraoperatively if needed or resected if an AGA flap cannot be positioned appropriately or accommodated when the posterior

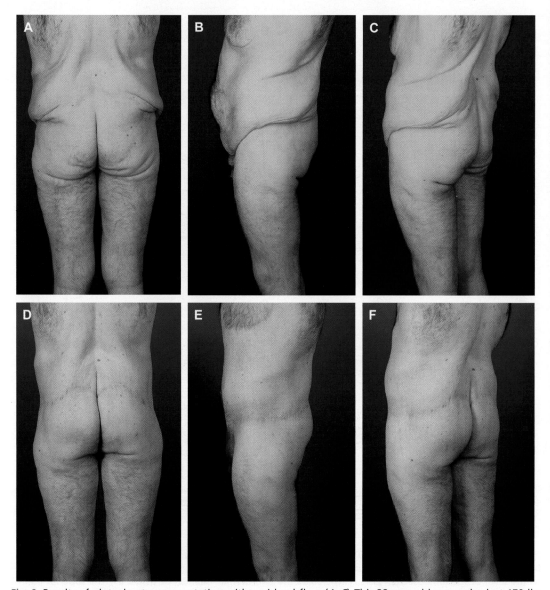

Fig. 9. Results of gluteal auto-augmentation with an island flap. (*A–C*) This 28-year-old man, who lost 170 lbs through diet and exercise, illustrates the loss of gluteal volume typical of MWL patients who achieve a normal BMI. (*D–F*) Postoperative views 10 months after the patient had an island flap augmentation at the time of CBL. In the same surgery he also had a mastopexy, medial thigh lift, and brachioplasty. Although the amount of volume added with the island flap is not great, he would have had significantly flattened buttocks after a CBL if the flap were not part of the procedure. Although high, the point of maximum gluteal projection is characteristic of most men.

CBL or upper and lower buttock lift flaps are brought together. Should there be any concern about tissue perfusion, excessive tension on the CBL closure, or inability to close the flaps over the gluteal tissue mound, the auto-augmentation should be abandoned so as not to compromise the safety of the lower body lift.

Complications

Complications directly related to AGA in 27 patients who have had the procedure in association with CBL performed by two authors (RFC and VLY) are shown in Table 1. No complications were major. The incidences do not seem to be significantly different from (and may be lower than) complications reported for CBL alone. For CBLs, the reported rates of delayed wound healing, epidermolysis, or skin necrosis range widely between 0% and 77%, with overall complication rates in the range of 10% to 80%.

Delayed wound healing is among the most common complications following CBL, and

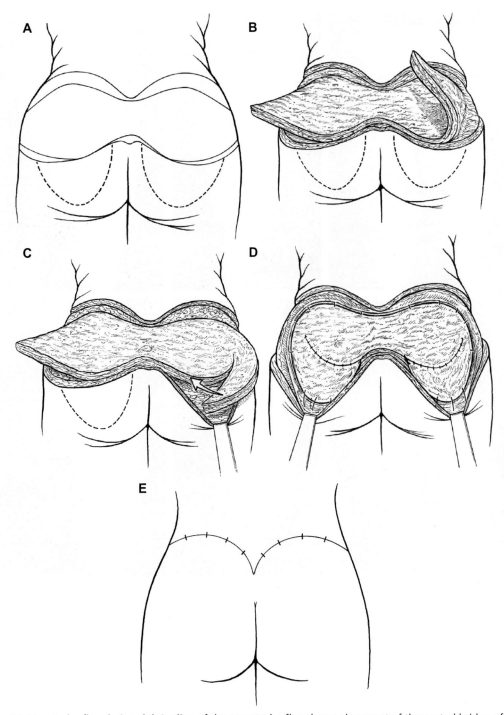

Fig. 10. Moustache flap design. (*A*) Outline of the moustache flap shows placement of the central bridge of tissue and lateral flap extensions, or handlebars. (*B*) The flap is de-epithelialized, and the moustache handlebars are elevated from the fascia. (*C*) The handlebars are rotated medially, any excess lateral tissue is trimmed off, and the flap is imbricated to itself laterally to prevent trochanteric fullness. (*D*) The rotated flaps are fixed centrally to the gluteal fascia with #1 Vicryl Plus and imbricated to create an anatomic mound of tissue. (*E*) A closed moustache flap with sparse stapling. (*From* Centeno RF. Autologous gluteal augmentation with circumferential body lift in the massive weight loss and aesthetic patient. Clin Plast Surg 2006;33:486; with permission.)

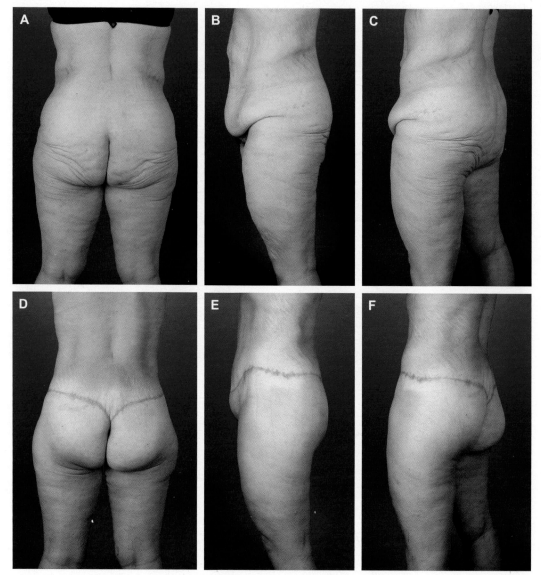

Fig. 11. (A–C) Preoperative views of a 35-year-old woman who lost 186 lbs (more than half her weight) after laparoscopic gastric bypass surgery. (D–F) Photographs taken 4 months after CBL with moustache flap for gluteal autoaugmentation. She also had a mastopexy, axilloplasty, and brachioplasty in the same surgery, followed 3 months later by an extended thighplasty and placement of breast implants. Some asymmetry of the buttocks is evident, but the patient is pleased with her surgical results.

minor delayed wound healing occurred in 6 of 25 patients undergoing AGA with CBL; however, this frequency is similar for patients undergoing CBL alone. Most patients who undergo gluteal augmentation with a flap have experienced MWL, and their history makes them more likely to be at greater risk for surgical complications than are patients who seek aesthetic gluteal contouring. Nonetheless, the undermining of the inferior CBL flap and tension on the closure is greater when AGA is added. This can lead to wound-healing problems, especially in the central aspect of

the incision, which is the "watershed" region of tissue perfusion.

The robust vascularization of an AGA flap and limitation of flap dissection to no more than two contiguous angiosomes seem to provide good flap perfusion and viability. One case of minor flap necrosis among our patients likely resulted from an excessively long "handlebar" lateral extension of the moustache flap into the "posterior-intercostal" angiosome described by Taylor [24]. Because this lateral extension is undermined to allow superomedial transposition of both halves of the moustache

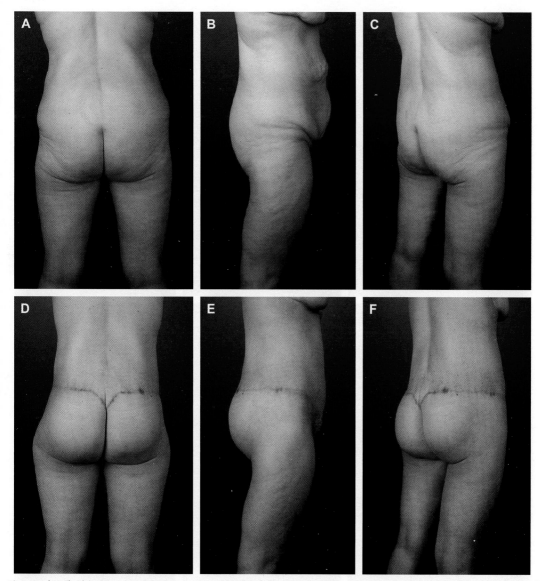

Fig. 12. (*A–C*) This 32-year-old woman lost 125 lbs following laparoscopic gastric bypass surgery. The loss of gluteal volume is particularly evident on the oblique view. (*D–F*) Six months after a CBL plus moustache flap, in addition to a mastopexy, axilloplasty, and brachioplasty. The improvement in gluteal contour is significant.

flap, the "two adjacent angiosomes" limitation of perforator flap perfusion may have been exceeded.

Careful preoperative planning to avoid overresection and beginning with conservatively sized flaps are helpful in preventing serious wound-healing problems, skin necrosis, and dehiscence. Although this may limit the quality and esthetics of a surgeon's early results, significantly better outcomes can be achieved after more experience is gained.

Large, clinically significant seromas that are due to dead space can be reduced by putting drains in the most dependent portion of the gluteal pockets. Quilting sutures are used routinely now to minimize dead space. Doxycycline sclerosis is the procedure of choice for managing postoperative seroma or excessive drain output in patients who have undergone CBL. Tissue sealants are not used because of cost considerations and the absence of convincing data regarding their effectiveness. As the collective experience with sealant products continues to accumulate, they may play a role in the management of seromas in patients undergoing CBL with or without AGA.

Anorectal hypersensitivity or maceration due to overexposure of the anus occurred in two of our patients who underwent AGA plus CBL. In both cases, the problem was self-limited as the expected skin laxity relapse and skin creep occurred. Until this

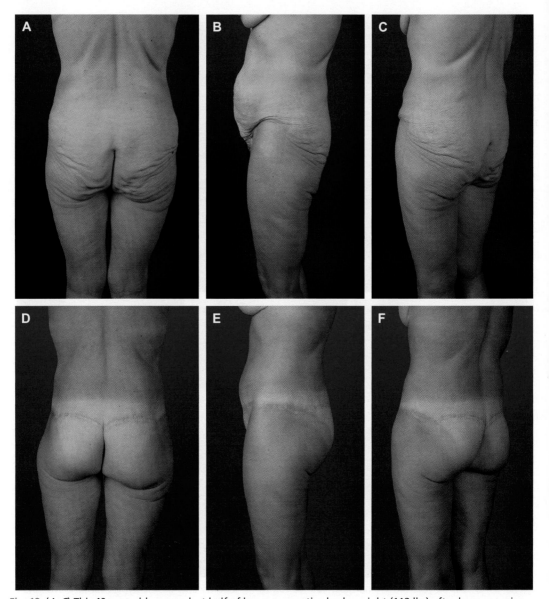

Fig. 13. (*A–C*) This 49-year-old woman lost half of her preoperative body weight (112 lbs) after laparoscopic gastric bypass surgery and ended up with a BMI of 20 kg/m² but significant skin laxity, which is worse in the right buttock. (*D–F*) Postoperative photos taken 14 months after a CBL plus moustache flap, mons reduction, mastopexy with breast auto-augmentation, axilloplasty, brachioplasty, and umbilicoplasty. Her low BMI and the absence of residual subcutaneous fat would have contributed to extreme buttock flattening if she had a CBL without auto-augmentation. The bikini worn by the patient covers her low CBL incision.

problem resolves, it can be managed with topical anesthetics (eg, Anusol), skin protectants, "donut" cushions for sitting, frequent positional changes, a high-fiber diet, sitz baths, and "baby wipes" for cleansing the area. Patient reassurance about the temporary nature of the problem is imperative.

Autologous fat transfer

The efficacy of autologous fat transfer in esthetic surgery has been contested vigorously, and the debate continues because of the lack of cost-effective and objective methods for measuring the viability of transferred autologous fat in vivo. In vitro studies have demonstrated that fat can survive the harvesting process, but the literature is inconclusive about the optimal approaches to the procurement, processing, and transferring of fat. Nonetheless, more and more surgeons have found that autologous fat transfer is clinically effective and can play an important role in body contouring.

Table 1: Complications of autologous gluteal augmentation with circumferential body lift for 27 patients

Complication	N (%)
Minor delayed wound healing	6 (22)
Superficial wound dehiscence	4 (15)
Major wound dehiscence	2 (7)
Infection	2 (7)
Temporary anal overexposure	2 (7)
Seroma requiring drainage	1 (4)
AGA flap malposition	1 (4)
Minor fat necrosis	1 (4)
Major fat necrosis	0
Skin necrosis	0
DVT or PE	0
Pressure sores	0
Long-term palpability	0

Abbreviations: DVT, deep vein thrombosis; PE, pulmonary embolism.

Autologous fat transfer for gluteal augmentation was reported first by Chajchir and colleagues [32] in 1990. Since then, multiple reports have verified the clinical efficacy of transferred fat for this application. Fat is harvested typically with liposuction cannulas using low-level suction (18–22 mm Hg). A sterile trap retains the fat, which is processed by adding antibiotics and by removing infranatant tumescent fluid and supranatant oil. Various methods for processing fat include centrifuging the fat at 2000 to 3000 revolutions per minute for 3 to 5 minutes, straining in a sieve, or using commercially available processing syringes. Transfer is accomplished with a blunt-tipped injection cannula or a small liposuction cannula. Multiple planes and passes are used to deliver the fat in aliquots to ensure even distribution in proximity to a blood supply. Successful use of syringes in the range of 1 to 30 mL has been reported [13,14,19,33,34]. Most investigators state that 50% to 100% of fat survives transfer, although estimation methods are vague [35].

Aggressive lumbosacral liposuction, in conjunction with judicious liposuction of the flanks, back, trochanteric area, medial thighs, anterior thighs, and abdomen, has been used synergistically to improve gluteal contour [13]. Liposuction of the infragluteal fold generally is contraindicated because of the supportive function of tissues in this area, and only minimal, careful liposuction should be performed in this area if an inharmonious tissue excess truly exists. Compression garment use is variable, but compression does seem helpful for avoiding fluid accumulation in the lumbosacral area. Patients should avoid sitting—except for going to the bathroom—for 1 to 2 weeks to minimize fat resorption as much as possible.

Patient satisfaction with fat transfer for gluteal augmentation is perceived to be high, despite the lack of systematic documentation in most published reports [13,14,33–36]. At the same time, however, reported combined major and minor complication rates have ranged from none to 52% and include seromas, infection, skin necrosis, contour irregularities, and sciatic nerve neurapraxia. Despite this complication profile, the frequency of complications tends to decline with growing surgeon experience. As an example, Bruner and colleagues [35] reported that 45% of their cases developed seroma that required aspiration, but that the number declined to 2% for more recent cases.

We believe that this trend applies to most surgeons as they gain experience with fat transfer and procedures become more refined. Fat transfer compares favorably with implant augmentation with respect to esthetics, but it seems to have a better safety profile than implants. In the United States, fat transfer has emerged as the leading technique for cosmetic gluteal contouring. Its application in MWL patients is increasing, but it is unclear whether its full potential will be realized. Several issues remain that may limit applicability in this population: the lack of enough available fat to overcome severe volume loss and skin laxity in MWL patients who have reached a low BMI; practical sequencing with excisional procedures because fat transfer is labor intensive; and the impact of compression from sitting on the resorption of fat if combined with excisional procedures that require supine postoperative positioning (eg, abdominoplasty and CBL).

Adjunctive excisional techniques for gluteal enhancement

The authors' collective experience with gluteal contouring and augmentation in the population that has experienced MWL suggests that no single technique is applicable to all gluteal deformities. The wide spectrum of deformities demands an individualized approach to each patient. Adjunctive excisional techniques at the time of autologous augmentation or CBL—or as a staged procedure in the most severe cases—often are necessary to obtain an optimal outcome. For some patients, skin excess or laxity in the posterior thigh, medial thigh, and infragluteal fold cannot be corrected fully with AGA or CBL. Furthermore, the orientation of the excision in a buttock lift may negatively affect the correction of skin laxity of the buttock proper. An infragluteal diamond lift is useful for enhancing this esthetic feature and achieving the 45°

downward-sloping angle at the junction between the infragluteal fold and the intergluteal crease.

The posterior thigh lift with dermotuberal anchoring, described by Gonzalez [37], is useful in contouring the posterior thigh and residual buttock ptosis at the time of CBL, provided that flap or implant augmentation is not performed. If autologous tissue or implant augmentation is incorporated into a CBL, it seems prudent to stage a posterior thigh lift as a secondary procedure, because it can involve significant undermining of the buttock skin. In contrast, the posterior thigh lift may be beneficial at the time of fat transfer, which requires no undermining. The orientation of the upper buttock lift excisions proposed by Gonzalez [37] may help to correct some gluteal esthetic unit deformities (eg, creating a sacral triangle), but its efficacy and safety have not been substantiated in the literature.

The "inverted dart" modification of the posterior CBL incision is another useful maneuver for improving gluteal esthetics [20,29]. It locates the incision between gluteal esthetic units and is a powerful tool for shortening and stabilizing the length of the intergluteal crease. A long intergluteal crease is not esthetically pleasing and can be a preexisting deformity in many patients who have experienced MWL. It also may be a surgically induced deformity caused by aggressive buttock lifting or by a medially rotated lifting vector.

Alloplastic implant augmentation techniques

As demand for gluteal enhancement has grown, so has the authors' clinical experience with the various forms of alloplastic and autologous augmentation. For MWL patients, gluteal implant designs have limitations, especially as a primary treatment for pronounced platypygia. Many patients who have experienced MWL lack sufficient fat or tissue volume to pad an implant, and their skin can be thin, which might make them more susceptible to implant migration, extrusion, palpability, or visibility. No literature has appeared about the use of gluteal implants in patients who have experienced MWL. Although implant augmentation can enhance gluteal esthetics successfully, the wide acceptance of this technique in the United States remains doubtful because the types of implants available are limited to silicone elastomer, and complications are not uncommon [35]. Despite this, augmentation with implants may still be applicable in certain subsets of carefully selected and well-informed patients, and some familiarity with implant procedures is important. The positioning of gluteal implants is illustrated in Fig. 14.

Submuscular

Submuscular implantation is easy to perform. The implant is covered by the gluteus maximus muscle, thus reducing the risk for implant visibility. Disadvantages include a point of maximal projection being created at a level that is too high (eg, a "shelf butt" or a potential "double bubble" effect). More serious complications include seromas (most common), wound dehiscence (second most common), implant migration, capsular contracture, implant extrusion or infection, compartment syndrome, or sciatica; however, the frequencies of complications are difficult to find in the literature [35].

With this technique, placement of an implant is limited by the anatomy of the sciatic nerve. The inferior extent of the submuscular dissection is at the level of the greater trochanters, which corresponds to the anatomic level at which the sciatic nerve exits from below the piriformis muscle. If the implant migrates below this level because of overdissection or inaccurate implant placement, symptoms of sciatic nerve compression are more likely. Submuscular placement of the implant and its proximity to the sciatic nerve also are likely responsible for the increased level of postoperative pain reported by patients receiving submuscular implants. Nonetheless, this technique probably will continue to play a role in gluteal augmentation in male patients. The short anthropometric shape of the male pelvis typically produces a point of maximum projection that is slightly higher than in women. The more superior placement required for submuscular implants translates to a favorable esthetic in male patients with a short buttock or female patients with superior third volume deficiency.

Intramuscular

Intramuscular gluteal augmentation with implants appears to achieve an esthetically pleasing result with minimal irregularities [11,38]. One reported series, by Vergara and Amezcua [12], showed a complication rate of 10% in 160 patients, including seromas (4%), asymmetry (2.6%), capsular contracture (2%), overcorrection (0.66%), and implant rupture (0.66%). The only series from the United States was reported by Mendieta [11], who had a 30% frequency of wound dehiscence before adopting a different incision [38]. An advantage of intramuscular implantation is that the anatomy of the sciatic nerve does not limit implant placement (Fig. 14B), although the dissection is challenging and risks shredding of the muscle. The lateral dissection of the muscle is critical because this is an area where the implant may move from the intramuscular plane to the subcutaneous plane, with its attendant consequences. Furthermore, from an esthetic

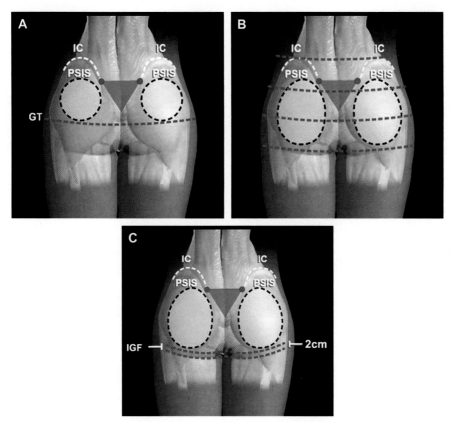

Fig. 14. Gluteal implant locations for (*A*) submuscular, (*B*) intramuscular, and (*C*) subfascial procedures. GT, greater trochanter; IC, iliac crest; IGF, infragluteal fold. (*From* Centeno RF, Young VL. Clinical anatomy in aesthetic gluteal body contouring surgery. Clin Plast Surg 2006;33:350; with permission.)

standpoint, the intramuscular technique places the implant in the middle of the buttock. If projection is needed in the superior or inferior third of the buttock, the final gluteal shape with intramuscular implants looks peculiar on lateral view. Despite these drawbacks, this technique may play a role in patients who have little adipose tissue in the gluteal region where subfascial implantation would produce palpability or visibility of the implant.

Subfascial

The subfascial approach to gluteal implantation was developed to solve the problems mentioned above with the other techniques [9]. As described by de la Peña and colleagues [39], the subfascial plane is undermined to raise the gluteal aponeurosis covering the anterior two thirds of the gluteus medius and maximus muscles. This dissection maintains the muscle integrity and allows it to be used as a platform for the implant. Once the implant is placed, the aponeurosis provides anatomic covering and contouring. Although this technique is limited by the anatomy, it is easy to perform. The results are reproducible, and subfascial placement produces a good esthetic outcome when lower pole volume

is desired, although implant palpability and visibility remain problems. In de la Pena's [9] report on 48 patients who had subfascial augmentation between 1990 and 1998, 85% believed that the result exceeded their expectations of an esthetically pleasing outcome. Complications included one implant contamination (2%), one pressure sore at the site requiring removal of the implant, and one seroma. In the United States, however, Bruner and colleagues [35] reported that 51% of patients receiving subfascial implants had at least one complication. Additional considerations include the learning curve associated with any new procedure, which may be a bit steeper because the dissection follows lines that are not on a natural anatomic plane. In addition, some special instruments are required, such as lighted retractors and a "calf dissector."

Technique selection and decision algorithm

Selection of a technique for gluteal contouring in MWL patients begins by classifying the deformity and evaluating the status of the subcutaneous adipose tissue in the gluteal region and the surrounding areas of the abdomen, flanks, back, hips, and

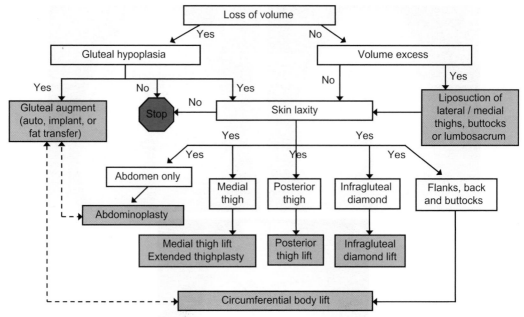

Fig. 15. MWL gluteal-contouring algorithm.

lower extremities. The MWL gluteal contouring algorithm (Fig. 15) illustrates the preferred choices for gluteal contouring under various conditions, depending on the deformities present. If there is a loss of tissue volume, skin laxity, and buttock ptosis, a CBL is the best option. Volume excess in areas surrounding the buttocks does not preclude the coexistence of gluteal hypoplasia, which is common in patients who have experienced MWL. In these cases, gluteal augmentation may be incorporated with the CBL, and adjunctive liposuction may be necessary.

High complication rates associated with various forms of implant augmentation have relegated these procedures to the last resort for our MWL patients. The safest results are obtained with autologous tissues, either as a flap or as transferred fat. Adjunctive excisional procedures also may be needed to address the thighs and infragluteal area; these can be performed simultaneously or in a staged fashion to refine results.

Summary

Gluteal contouring and augmentation techniques are requested often by patients who have experienced MWL and want something done about the "flat butt" that followed weight loss. These patients must be informed during consultation that this platypygia will likely be made even worse by a CBL unless volume is added to the gluteal region. Moreover, some patients who require an abdominoplasty, rather than a CBL, to address their skin excess also may suffer from gluteal hypoplasia that

requires volume addition and contouring. Several options are available in the MWL body contouring armamentarium: AGA with CBL, a buttock-flank lift, autologous fat transfer, adjunctive excisional techniques, and, less commonly, implant augmentation. As we continue to advance in our understanding of the deformities that affect our patients who have experienced MWL, these techniques undoubtedly will be refined. We also will become wiser in choosing the most appropriate techniques for different kinds of patients, which should lead to fewer complications and improved esthetic outcomes.

References

[1] Babuccu O, Gozil R, Ozmen S, et al. Gluteal region morphology: the effect of weight gain and aging. Aesthetic Plast Surg 2002;26(2):130–3.

[2] Da Rocha RP. Surgical anatomy of the gluteal region's subcutaneous screen and its use in plastic surgery. Aesthetic Plast Surg 2001;25:140–4.

[3] Toth MJ, Tchernof A, Sites CK, et al. Menopause-related changes in body fat distribution. Ann NY Acad Sci 2000;904:502–6.

[4] Kopelman PG. The effects of weight loss treatments on upper and lower body fat. Int J Obes 1997;21:619–25.

[5] Ferretti A, Giampiccolo P, Cavalli A, et al. Expiratory flow limitation and orthopnea in massively obese subjects. Chest 2001;119:1401–8.

[6] Watson RA, Pride NB. Postural changes in lung volumes and respiratory resistance in subjects with obesity. J Appl Physiol 2005;98:512–7.

[7] Fabris de Souza SA, Faintuch J, Valezi AC, et al. Postural changes in morbidly obese patients. Obes Surg 2005;15:1013–6.

[8] Giusti V, Gasteyger C, Suter M, et al. Gastric banding induces negative remodeling in the absence of secondary hyperparathyroidism: potential role of serum c telopeptides for follow-up. Int J Obes (Lond) 2005;29(12):1429–35.

[9] de la Peña JA. Subfascial technique for gluteal augmentation. Aesthetic Surgery Journal 2004; 24:265–73.

[10] Gonzalez-Ulloa M. Gluteoplasty: a ten-year report. Aesthetic Plast Surg 1991;15:85–91.

[11] Mendieta CG. Gluteoplasty. Aesthetic Surgery Journal 2003;23(6):441–55.

[12] Vergara R, Amezcua H. Intramuscular gluteal implants: fifteen years' experience. Aesthetic Surgery Journal 2003;23(2):86–91.

[13] Cárdenas-Camarena L, Lacouture AM, Tobar-Losada A. Combined gluteoplasty: liposuction and lipoinjection. Plast Reconstr Surg 1999; 104(5):1524–31.

[14] Valero de Pedroza L. Fat transplantation to the buttocks and legs for aesthetic enhancement or correction of deformities: long-term results of large volumes of fat transplant. Dermatol Surg 2000;26(12):1145–9.

[15] Pascal JF, Le Louarn C. Remodeling bodylift with high lateral tension. Aesthetic Plast Surg 2002; 26:223–30.

[16] Regnault P, Daniel R. Secondary thigh-buttock deformities after classical techniques: prevention and treatment. Clin Plast Surg 1984;11(3):505–16.

[17] Cuenca-Guerra R, Quezada J. What makes buttocks beautiful? A review and classification of the determinants of gluteal beauty and the surgical techniques to achieve them. Aesthetic Plast Surg 2004;28:340–7.

[18] Centeno RF, Young VL. Clinical anatomy in aesthetic gluteal body contouring surgery. Clin Plast Surg 2006;33:347–58.

[19] Roberts TL III, Weinfeld AB, Bruner TW, et al. "Universal" and ethnic ideals of beautiful buttocks are best obtained by autologous micro fat grafting and liposuction. Clin Plast Surg 2006; 33:371–94.

[20] Centeno RF. Gluteal Aesthetic Unit classification: a tool to improve outcomes in body contouring. Aesthetic Surgery Journal 2006;26:200–8.

[21] Matarasso A, Wallach G. Abdominal contour surgery: treating all aesthetic units, including the mons pubis. Aesthetic Surgery Journal 2001;21:111–9.

[22] Drake RL, Wayne V, Mitchell AWM. Gray's anatomy for students. Philadelphia: Elsevier, Churchill, Livingstone; 2005.

[23] Strauch B, Vasconez LO, Hall-Findlay EJ. Grabb's encyclopedia of flaps. 2nd edition. Philadelphia: Lippincott-Raven; 1988.

[24] Taylor GI. The angiosomes of the body and their supply to perforator flaps. Clin Plast Surg 2003; 30:331–42.

[25] Mendieta CG. Classification system for gluteal evaluation. Clin Plast Surg 2006;33:333–46.

[26] Gonzalez M, Guerrerosantos J. Deep planed torso-abdominoplasty combined with buttocks pexy. Aesthetic Plast Surg 1997;21(4):245–53.

[27] Guerrerosantos J. Secondary hip-buttock-thigh plasty. Clin Plast Surg 1984;11(3):491–503.

[28] Pitanguy I. Surgical reduction of the abdomen, thighs and buttocks. Surg Clin North Am 1971; 51:479–89.

[29] Centeno RF. Autologous gluteal augmentation with circumferential body lift in the massive weight loss and aesthetic patient. Clin Plast Surg 2006;33:479–96.

[30] Young VL, Centeno RF. The role of large-volume liposuction and other adjunctive procedures. In: Rubin JP, Matarasso A, editors. Aesthetic surgery after massive weight loss. Philadelphia: Elsevier Saunders; 2007. p. 167–87.

[31] Colwell AS, Borud LJ. Autologous gluteal augmentation after massive weight loss: aesthetic analysis and role of the superior gluteal artery perforator flap. Plast Reconstr Surg 2007;119: 345–56.

[32] Chajchir A, Benzaquen I, Wexler E, et al. Fat injection. Aesthetic Plast Surg 1990;14:127–36.

[33] Roberts TL, Toledo LS, Baden AZ. Augmentation of the buttocks by micro fat grafting. Aesthetic Surgery Journal 2001;21:311–9.

[34] Murillo WL. Buttock augmentation: case studies of fat injection monitored by magnetic resonance imaging. Plast Reconstr Surg 2004;114: 1606–14.

[35] Bruner TW, Roberts TL III, Nguyen K. Complications of buttocks augmentation: diagnosis, management, and prevention. Clin Plast Surg 2006; 33:449–66.

[36] Peren PA, Gomez JB, Guerrerosantos J, et al. Gluteus augmentation with fat grafting. Aesthetic Plast Surg 2000;24:412–7.

[37] Gonzalez R. Buttocks lifting: how and when to use medial, lateral, lower, and upper lifting techniques. Clin Plast Surg 2006;33:467–78.

[38] Mendieta CG. Intramuscular gluteal augmentation technique. Clin Plast Surg 2006;33: 423–34.

[39] De la Peña JA, Rubio OV, Cano JP, et al. Subfascial gluteal augmentation. Clin Plast Surg 2006; 33:405–22.

ELSEVIER SAUNDERS

CLINICS IN
PLASTIC
SURGERY

Clin Plastic Surg 35 (2008) 93

Editorial Commentary

The authors of the last three articles demonstrate the gamut of philosophy on buttocks augmentation in body lift surgery. Centeno and Young have been instrumental in developing auto-augmentation flap techniques that they feel have led to improved buttocks projection. Although these authors are able to attain excellent results, I use my editor's prerogative to voice a differing opinion. It is my experience from dealing with buttocks flap auto-augmentations that they can be very difficult to master, they increase operating time by at least 45 minutes in the best of hands, and in inexperienced hands they can lead to bizarre buttocks contour. Although Centeno and Young report a very low complication rate, in my experience other surgeons are not so adept. Serious complications of skin or fat necrosis, chronic seromas resistant to treatment, infections, and sepsis have all occurred.

Richter's technique may seem to be somewhat similar to buttocks flap auto-augmentation, but it is not. In his technique he leaves behind all the fat that is deep to the superficial fascial system of the buttocks and shapes that fat with sutures to create projection. There are no fat or dermal flaps created in his technique. I believe Richter's technique is much safer and more reproducible when compared with auto-augmentation buttocks flaps, especially for beginning surgeons. Capella, similar to us, does not espouse or use auto-augmentation and he attains excellent results also.

Overall it is our feeling that fat injections should be the preferred method of increasing buttocks projection in patients who have undergone massive weight loss. One should "never say never" to flap auto-augmentation, but it should be reserved for special circumstances.

plasticsurgery.theclinics.com

doi:10.1016/j.cps.2007.10.015

ELSEVIER
SAUNDERS

CLINICS IN
PLASTIC
SURGERY

Clin Plastic Surg 35 (2008) 95–104

Lipoabdominoplasty

Ramón Vila-Rovira, MD

- Material and method
- Anesthetic protocol
- Preoperative protocol
- Surgical technique
  Fundamentals of the technique
  Performing the procedure
- Postoperative protocol
- Results

Clinical cases
Complications
- Discussion and commentaries
  Advantages
  Disadvantages
- Summary
- References

Abdominoplasty and liposuction are common surgeries, but when done simultaneously, as is happening more often, they represent a challenge for many surgeons. To make these combined procedures safe, the periumbilical perforator vessels must be preserved to prevent ischemia and avoid distress of the abdominal flap [1].

Early abdominoplasties only removed the skin and subcutaneous tissue through vertical incisions. Before the 1970s, body-contouring surgery was limited to the traditional open dermolipectomies with excision of skin and fat *en bloc* as described by Pitanguy [2]. In 1960, as greater exposure of the body became more fashionable, abdominoplasties with horizontal suprapubic incisions were described. Callia [3], in response to demand for shorter scars and better outcomes, described an original method with smaller incisions and faster recoveries.

These procedures produce two possible unesthetic sequelae. One is the scar, which is difficult to hide, and the other is the redundant tissue at both ends of the scar. Because of these problems, research on subcutaneous surgery or "collapsing surgery" began.

Subcutaneous surgery, or closed technique, was initiated by Schrudde [4] in 1972, followed by Fischer and Fischer [5] in 1977, and Kesselring and Meyer [6] in 1978. They basically used a uterine curette for the extraction of fat without scissor dissection of the subcutaneous fat. However, most of their cases required revision surgeries and few surgeons could reproduce this technique with a low incidence of complications.

In early 1980, Illouz [7] described liposuction for body contouring. With the use of cannulae, the concept of tunneling rapidly displaced existing techniques because tunnelling was easy to reproduce and resulted in fewer complications. Illouz [8,9] popularized liposuction, changing forever the concepts of body contouring and consequently the future of abdominoplasties.

Since then, many related papers have been published describing various liposuction techniques. In 1983, Fournier and Otteni [10] introduced his dry technique liposuction. In 1986, Hakme [11] and Wilkinson and Swartz [12] combined liposuction with partial abdominoplasty. The author and colleagues in 1985 [13] described the combination of liposuction and abdominoplasty, which was further described in 1987 in *Liposuction in Plastic and Aesthetic Surgery* [14]. This was followed by Matarasso's 1991 and 1995 anatomical studies [15,16] describing the safety areas for combined lipoabdominoplasty.

In 1992, Illouz [17] described an abdominoplasty after an abdominal liposuction, thus creating

Institut Vila-Rovira, Centro Médico Teknon, C/Vilana, 12 Despacho 128, 08022 Barcelona, Spain
E-mail address: dr@vilarovira.com

doi:10.1016/j.cps.2007.09.002

the concept of mesh undermining. He was followed by Shestak [18] (1999) with an article about liposuction combined with partial resection of suprapubic skin without undermining.

Avelar [19,20] in 1999 and 2000 added the excision of skin with submammary incisions to address the issue of excision of supraumbilical skin with or without video-endoscopic plication of the rectus muscles.

Saldaña [21,22] in 2001 and 2003 described the complete liposuction of the abdomen combined with a classical abdominoplasty with selective undermining of the flaps with transposition of the umbilicus, creating the term lipoabdominoplasty, a procedure that is now routine.

This article describes extensive liposuction with minimal abdominoplasty, a technique developed by the author and colleagues at Institut Vila-Rovira. The technique represents another step in the evolution of liposuction procedures.

Obesity is a chronic multifactorial disease considered by the World Health Organization as the "twentieth-century epidemic." It is closely related to genetic, social, environmental, neurological, cultural, and biological factors and unhealthy eating habits throughout life [23].

To determine if an individual male or female is considered obese, we at the Institut Vila-Rovira use the body mass index (BMI) [23]. A BMI of 25 or less is considered normal; a BMI of 25 to 30 is considered overweight; a BMI between 30 and 35 represents pathologic obesity; a BMI of 35 to 40 represents grave obesity; and a BMI of more than 40 represents morbid obesity [23].

This article describes a surgical alternative for those patients with a BMI of 30 to 35. This procedure, which the author and colleagues at the Institut Vila-Rovira call extensive liposuction with minimal abdominoplasty (ELMA), preserves the safety of the conventional lipoabdominoplasties.

Material and method

Clinicians at the Institut Vila-Rovira have used the ELMA procedure to treat 48 patients between 26 and 48 years old with an average weight of 100 kg and a BMI between 30 and 35.

In all cases, liposuction of between 6 and 24 L and minimal dissection abdominoplasty was done. In cases of grave obesity, bariatric surgery was recommended, followed by postbariatric plastic surgery.

Anesthetic protocol

Before the procedure, a preoperative evaluation by an anesthesiologist is important for the selection and care of these patients. American Society of Anesthesiologists (ASA) class 1 and 2 anesthetics are acceptable with strict monitoring.

BMI should be less than 35 with preoperative laboratory tests according to the recommendations of the Confederation of Latin American Societies of Anesthesiologists.

Hematocrit and hemoglobin, glucose, liver panel, coagulation profile and serology plus electrocardiogram, chest radiograph, and cardiovascular evaluation are obtained.

Measures to prevent pulmonary embolism should be instituted, especially in those patients with moderate or high risk, such as patients older than 40 years, those that will undergo prolonged procedures (more than 4 hours), those using contraceptives, those with chronic or malignant diseases, and those with a history of deep vein thrombosis or pulmonary embolism. Those measures will be discussed below.

Intraoperative fluid management should be strict because of "third spacing" of fluids and colloids with volume shifting similar to that occurring in surgical trauma (autoresuscitation).

The hourly intravenous administration of saline solution should be equal to the basal requirement (follow 4-2-1 rule, which is based on the relation between body weight and metabolic rate [Box 1]) plus the insensible losses (7 mL/kg). In a patient with a weight of 70 kg, the intravenous administration of saline solution should not be greater than 600 mL/h.

Infiltration with a modified Klein solution (3 L of saline plus 1 A of 1:1000 epinephrine) into the subcutaneous tissue will allow its permanence in the subcutaneous tissue and its slow return to the systemic circulation. The patient typically gains weight in the first 12 hours, returning to the preoperative infiltration level in 48 hours.

Box 1: 4-2-1 Rule for intravenous administration of saline solution

- 4 mL/kg/h of saline solution for the first 10 kg of body weight
- Plus 2 mL/kg/h of saline solution for the next 10 kg of body weight
- Plus 1 mL/h of saline solution for every kilogram of body weight over 20 kg

Thus, in a hypothetical case of a 65-kg patient, clinicians should administer 40 mL/h of saline solution for the first 10 kg of body weight plus 20 mL/h for the next 10 kg of body weight and 45 mL/h for the remaining 45 kg. In total, 105 mL/h of saline solution (40+20+65) should be administered. For adults, this formula requires 6 mL/kg/h up to 20 kg and 1 mL/kg/h for every kg of body weight over 20 kg.

After the infiltration with Klein's modified solution, aspiration of the fat with the ELMA technique yields 80% fat and 20% fluids. Fluid and blood should be replaced according to the volume of aspirated fat (VAF), following established formulas in the tumescent technique:

- For aspirated volume of less than 2 L: Minor fluid is replaced at a 1:1 ratio, intravenous-fluid/VAF. Blood loss is compensated with the infusion of saline solution.
- For VAF of 3 to 5 L: Fluid is replaced at a 1:1 ratio, intravenous–saline-solution/VAF. Blood loss is replaced with colloid at a 1:1 ratio.
- For VAF of more than 6 L: Fluid is replaces at a 1:1 ratio, intravenous–saline-solution/VAF. Blood loss is replaced with packed red blood cells at a 1:1 ratio.

It is necessary to determine the blood loss during the procedure. If more than 30% of the circulating volume is lost (approximately 1500 mL of blood), red blood cell transfusion is necessary.

The acute loss of the red blood cell mass triggers compensatory mechanisms to increase oxygen transport, such as increased alveolar gas exchange, cardiac output, and oxygen affinity for the blood cells.

Hematocrit decreases in 2% to 3% 6 hours after infiltration and returns to its preoperative levels 48 hours after the procedure. Hence, the hematocrit needs to be checked 2 days after surgery.

The critical level generally accepted is hemoglobin between 7 to 10 g/dL or a hematocrit of between 21% and 30%. It is best to avoid decreases of hematocrit below 30%. One unit of packed cells increases the hemoglobin 1 g/dL and the hematocrit 2% to 3%. It is important and necessary to determine the residual fluid volume (RFV), which is the infiltrated saline plus the intravenous fluids minus aspirated fat plus diuresis and drainage. This should be less than 70 mL/kg to avoid fluid overload and water toxicity, which can lead to such complications as pulmonary edema, dilutional hyponatremia, hemolysis, coagulopathies, and cardiovascular disturbances.

We at the Institut Vila-Rovira use amoxicillin-clavulanic - 1 unit/500 mg intravenously every 8 hours for 1 day and amoxicillin-clavulanic - 1 tablet/500 mg every 8 hours for 7 days.

An equally important concern is the prevention of pulmonary embolism, which is the main cause of liposuction-related mortality in the United States (1:5000 liposuctions).

In October 1998, the American Society of Plastic Surgeons (ASPS) task force on pulmonary embolism issuing the following recommendations:

- Early ambulation is advised and should be started within the first 24 hours after surgery in a gradual fashion.
- Elastic bandages should be employed because they improve venous flow, although there is no clear evidence that they prevent pulmonary embolism.
- Sequential pressure of lower limbs should be applied because it increases blood flow and favors fibrinolytic activity.
- Heparin should be administered in low doses of 5000 units subcutaneously 2 hours before surgery and every 12 hours after, according to risk (Heparin is not generally used at Institut Vila-Rovira.)
- Low molecular weight heparin can be used in the first 24 hours postoperatively.
- Strict monitoring is important in the first 48 hours.

Preoperative protocol

The patient must be informed about the benefits and risks of surgery in sufficient detail to allow for true understanding. At the Institut Vila-Rovira, blood work, EKG with cardiovascular evaluation and chest radiograph, referral to the blood bank for donation of 400 mL of autologous blood 30 and 15 days before the scheduled procedure are all routine for this patient population. The autologous blood is administered to the patient after the procedure. Preoperative discussions are held to go over a number of issues. Patients are told about their recovery, which takes place at home for 3 weeks with progressive return to work in 3 or 4 weeks. The patient is also told to use pressure garments for 1 to 2 months and is advised about a postoperative nutritional program and a workout program with personal trainers.

Surgical technique

Fundamentals of the technique

The technique involves extensive circumferential liposuction with plication of the rectus abdominis muscles preserving the perforators and excision of redundant abdominal skin under general anesthesia.

After evaluation by the attending anesthesiologist in the holding room, the patient is transferred to the operating room where he or she is marked for the circumferential liposuction of the lower trunk and also marked for proposed areas of open excision on the anterior abdomen. The boundary to mark is a horizontal line from the scapular tips above to another upper gluteal one below, sparing the so called "Bermuda triangle" of Illouz, which is marked by a sacral midline and a horizontal line through the ischial tuberosities. Laterally, the lines extend to the axillary areas and the flanks. Anteriorly, the lines extend to the submammary level and inferiorly to the inguinal region and pubis, inclusive. The patient is also evaluated sitting down to assess those areas that require special attention for the circumferential liposuction. We also perform the "pinch" test and notice any depressions, hollows, scars, and similar imperfections. Last, we mark the area of redundant skin to be resected in the abdominoplasty with the elliptical design of the conventional abdominoplasty including umbilical transposition extending the ends of the wound to avoid "dog ears." The pubic area should always be lipoaspirated, an important detail. Finally, while visualizing the final result to determine how the skin retraction will affect the final outcome, we create traction on the skin inferiorly. Marks are modified accordingly.

Once the marking is finished, the patient is anesthetized in the supine position on a stretcher. After insertion of a Foley catheter, the patient is then transferred to the operating table in the prone position. Two pillows are placed between the breasts and the pubis to straighten the back and facilitate the liposuction maneuvers. The arms are placed forward and the head rests in a hollow head holder.

Surgery is performed in the main operating rooms of our clinic under general anesthesia, always with a hematocrit above 32, which is restored with two units of packed red blood cells when it decreases to 28 or 30.

The general anesthetic is always performed with alertness monitoring, pulse oximeter, capnometer, and diuresis monitoring through the Foley catheter.

The procedure is started on the back.

Performing the procedure

We use diluted iodine povidone and sterile disposable drapes. If marking is needed, we mark with sterile skin markers. With a #15 blade, we make 3-mm long incisions on the intergluteal fold at the level of S1, S2, S3, S4, and S5, and we place them in such a way that we divide the area into three zones. We proceed with the tumescent infiltration of the back with a solution made up of 2 mL of epinephrine for each 3 L of saline, maximum of 2 bags for 3 L, using the necessary amount and infusing it with a positive-pressure pump. We wait 15–20 minutes for adequate vasoconstriction, and we perform "six hands" liposuction on the back and flanks with three flexible 3-mm cannulae all the way out to the "floatation line" that corresponds to the mid-axillary line. This is where liposuction stops in each position. Then we perform a mechanical release to even up the subdermal irregularities with a spatula

cannula not connected to the suction machine. We close the wounds with 6-0 nylon and turn the patient to the supine position.

The patient is reprepped and draped, and the surgical team changes gowns and gloves. We place the anterior infiltration incisions (as many as needed) near the upper end of the abdominal skin ellipse to be resected. If necessary, we make two mid-submammary incisions. Through these incisions, we infuse the tumescent solution as we did on the other side.

After 20 minutes, we start the extensive liposuction of the abdomen, pubis, and lateral thoracic areas and the release for liposculpture. At this point, the anesthesiologist starts a line with hot fluids to maintain the temperature of the patient.

We perform the pinch test for symmetry and make the necessary corrections. It is important to perform the "tent" test (ie, raising the cannula while the cannula is under the dermis). The endpoint is the point where the cannula contour is clearly defined.

Once we complete the liposuction, we continue with the abdominoplasty using Avelar's techniques with minimal undermining, plication of the fascia with a #0 Vicryl running stitch back and forth, and the transposition of the umbilicus.

The undermining creates a tunnel that extends from the umbilicus to the xiphoid. We spare the perforators and preserve Scarpa's fascia to reduce bleeding and to provide uniform support to the thinned abdominal flap. The plication extends from pubis to xiphoid in two segments separated by the umbilicus.

The umbilicoplasty is performed next and we prefer the "star" technique. Lower abdominal closure is done in layers with 3-0 and 4-0 Vicryl and 4-0 and 5-0 nylon. We leave drains in for 2 to 7 days, depending on the output. We place an elastic binder to be used for 30 days. Postoperatively, the patient's blood is autotransfused. Patients remain in the hospital for 2 nights and are discharged according to their progress.

Postoperative protocol

These patients experience a slightly prolonged recovery period as compared with those recovering from conventional liposuctions of less than 5 L, but the careful technique used to preserve the blood vessels and nerves makes the recovery period acceptable.

The use of an elastic binder for 30 to 60 days is very important. We change dressings initially between days 2 and 7, and we prescribe 7 to 10 days of rest at home with minimal basic activities.

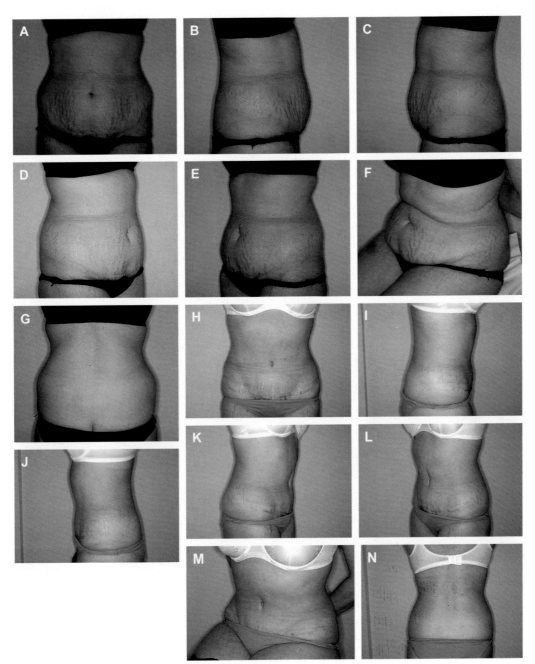

Fig. 1. (*A–G*) Before operation. (*H–N*) After operation.

On day 21, we remove all stitches and cover the scars with polyurethane because polyurethane's hypoxic effect prevents hypertrophic and keloid scars.

Simultaneously, the patient is enrolled in the Re-tone program, which is a postoperative 1-year program that includes physical and nutritional treatment. Follow-up and medical control are necessary after any esthetic, plastic, or reconstructive surgery. The goal is to achieve a fast recovery and optimize the outcome through four indispensable and fundamental principles:

- Control of medical and cicatricial variables
- Control of skin flacidity by means of massages and lymphatic drainage
- Control of nutrition
- Participation in personal physical exercise and recovery program

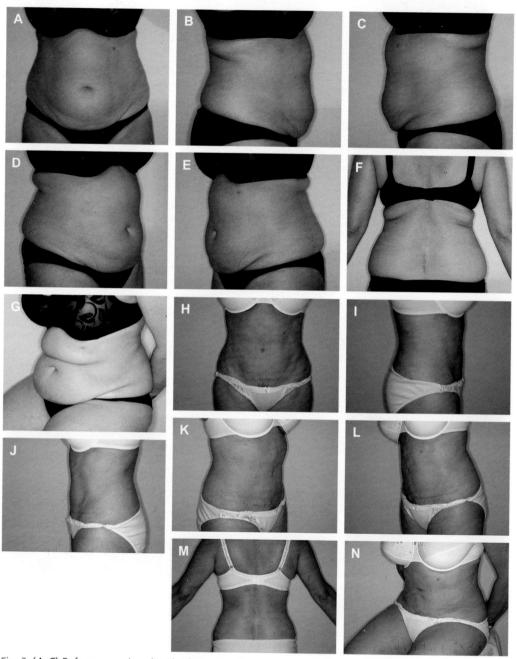

Fig. 2. (*A–G*) Before operation. (*H–N*) After operation.

Our personal physical exercise and recovery program, called the Re-tone program, emphasizes the neuromuscular recovery of the treated areas to restore the optimal motion of the hips, clavicles, and other parts of the body. In other words, it is designed to reactivate the muscles as soon as possible, to restore back posture and muscular tone, and to accelerate recovery in general. Other advantages are that it improves drainage of the treated area, restores respiratory volume, fosters control of the alimentary habits, and enhances the tone of the pelvic floor.

The purpose of the postoperative program and Re-tone "toning" is to maximize the effects of the surgery and make them last longer, therefore improving the physical shape, health, and self-image.

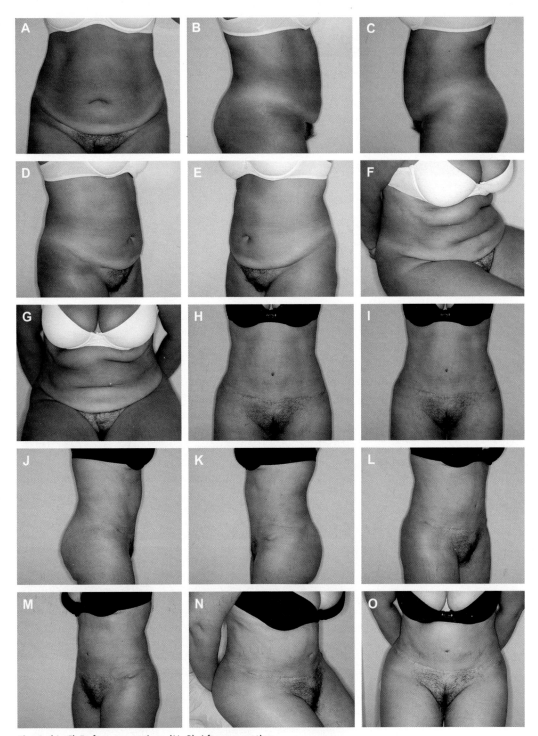

Fig. 3. (*A–G*) Before operation. (*H–O*) After operation.

This program can be accomplished in fractions of 3 months, but the patient is not discharged until 12 months have elapsed.

The treatments are provided by the surgeons, the physical therapists, the personal trainers, the nutritionists, and the dietary personnel.

This postoperative program is the best way to guarantee the outcome of the procedure and to maintain results. This program is most successful when the involved professionals are duly trained and totally committed to the patient. Therefore, continuous training is necessary.

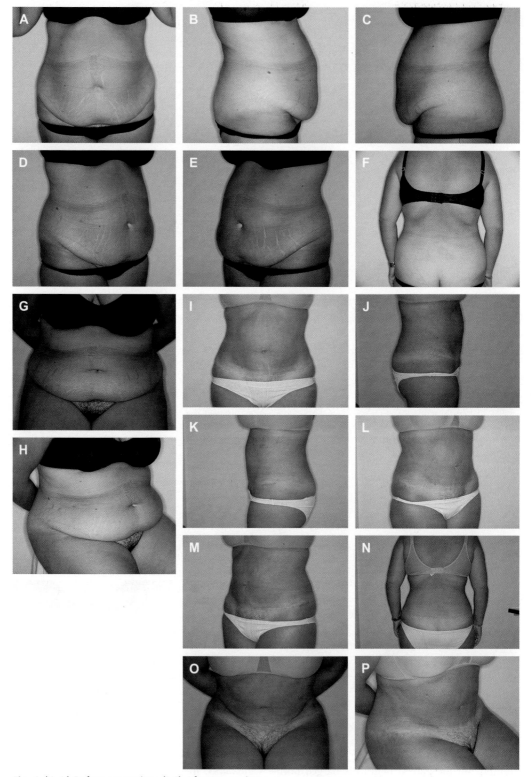

Fig. 4. (*A–H*) Before operation. (*I–P*) After operation.

Results

Clinical cases

Figs. 1–4 show preoperative and postoperative images. Globally considered, the outcomes reveal esthetic body changes, circumferential changes, and good outcome of the scars.

Complications

The well-systematized and careful procedures have resulted in a considerable reduction of complications:

- **Seromas—10%** [4]
- **Small areas of skin necrosis—10%** [4]
- **Hematomas—2%** [1]
- **Cutaneous irregularities—20%** [8]
- **Secondary miniliposuction—10%** [4]
- **Scar revisions—10%** [4]

Skin necroses occurred in difficult patients and were treated with silver sulfadiazine for 2 months and then revised.

Discussion and commentaries

Advantages

The advantages of the procedure include (1) better body-contour outcome thanks to the massive circumferential liposuction, (2) less morbidity because perforator vessels are spared and dead space eliminated, (3) a more natural result in obese patients who are difficult to treat with diets, and (4) preservation of suprapubic sensation.

Disadvantages

Disadvantages of the procedure include (1) greater morbidity due to the extensive nature of the procedure and large volume liposuction, (2) the need to have a complex and well-trained facility with adequate equipment and a systematic protocol, and (3) a long recovery due to the extent of liposuction.

Summary

Obese patients present more difficult challenges than those patients who are simply overweight or those with localized adiposity. The classical techniques do not satisfy the needs of obese patients, so alternative techniques, such as the one presented here, need to be considered. With this technique, we have noticed an improvement in the psychological and body image of these patients.

References

[1] Bostwick J III, Hartrampf F, Nahai F. The superiorly based rectus abdominis flap: predicting and enhancing its blood supply based on anatomic and clinical study. Plast Reconstr Surg 1988;81: 713.

[2] Pitanguy I. Trochanteric lipodystrophy. Plast Reconstr Surg 1964;34:280.

[3] Callia W. Contribuicao para o estudo da correcto cirurgico do abdome pendulo e globoso—Técnica original (disertation). Faculty of the Medical University of Sao Paulo, 1965.

[4] Schrudde J. Lipexeresis in the correction of local adiposity. First Congress of the International Society of Aesthetic and Plastic Surgeons. Rio de Janeiro, 1972.

[5] Fischer A, Fischer GM. Revised technique for cellulitis fat reduction in riding breeches deformity. Bull Int Acad Cosm Surg 1977;2:40–3.

[6] Kesselring UK, Meyer R. A suction curette for removal of excessive local deposits of subcutaneous fat. Plast Reconstr Surg 1978;62:305.

[7] Illouz YG. Une nouvelle techhnique pour les lipodysthrophies localices. Rev Chir Esth Franc 1980;6(19).

[8] Illouz YG. Reflexions apres 4 ans et demi d'experience et 800 cas de ma technique de lipolyse. Rev Chir Esth Franc 1981;6(24).

[9] Illouz YG. Body contouring by lipolisis: a 5-year experience with over 3000 cases. Plast Reconstr Surg 1983;72:591.

[10] Fournier PF, Otteni FM. Lipodissection in body sculpturing: the dry procedure. Plast Reconstr Surg 1983;72:598.

[11] Hakme F. Technical details in the liposuction associated with abdominoplasty. Rev Bras Cir 1985;75:331.

[12] Wilkinson TS, Swartz BE. Individual modification in body contour surgery: the limited abdoinoplasty. Plast Reconstr Surg 1986; 779–84.

[13] Vila-Rovira R, Serra Renom JM, Guinot A. Liposucción abdominal asociada a abdominoplastia. Cir Plást Iberolatinoamericana 1985;Vol. 4.

[14] Vila-Rovira R, Serra Renom JM. Liposucción en Cirugía Plástica y Estética. Liposucción abdominal combinada con abdominoplastia 1987;81.

[15] Matarasso A. Abdominolioplasty: a system of classification and treatment for combined abdominoplasty and suction assisted lipectomy. Aesthetic Plast Surg 1991;15:111–21.

[16] Matarasso A. Liposuction as an adjunct to a full abdominoplasty. Plast Reconstr Surg 1995;95: 829–36.

[17] Illouz YG. A new safe and aesthetc approach to suction abdominoplasty. Aesthetic Plast Surg 1992;16:237–45.

[18] Shestak KC. Marriage abdominoplasty expands the miniabdominoplasty concept. Plast Reconstr Surg 1999;103:120–35.

[19] Avelar JM. Uma nova técnica de abdoinoplastia-sistema vascular fechado de retalho subdérmico dobrado sobre si memo combinado com lipoaspiracao. Rev Bras Cir 1999;13: 3–20.

[20] Avelar JM. Abdominoplasty: a new technique without undermining and fat layer renoval. Arq Catarinense de Med 2000;29:147–9.

[21] Saldaña OR, De Souza Pinto EB, Matos WN Jr, et al. Lipoabdominoplasty without undermining. Aesthetic Surg J 2001;21:518–26.

[22] Saldaña OR. Lipoabdominoplasty with selective and safe undermining. Aesthetic Plast Surg 2003;27:322–7.

[23] Aly AS. Body contouring after massive weight loss. St Louis (MO): QMP; 2006. p. 4–6.

ELSEVIER
SAUNDERS

CLINICS IN
PLASTIC
SURGERY

Clin Plastic Surg 35 (2008) 105

Editorial Commentary

Before personally observing and evaluating the procedure that Dr. Vila-Rovira presents in his article, I was skeptical about its capability to improve lower truncal contour in patients who had undergone massive weight loss because it was my experience that circumferential excess in these patients is only amenable to circumferential excisional procedures. Additionally, large-volume liposuction can be difficult to use routinely in the highly litigious United States malpractice environment. I believe the reader can see that Vila-Rovira's technique obviously has merit, as evidenced by the results shown in the article. I believe it can be used in patients who have reasonable skin elasticity despite their weight loss; thus the selection criteria need to be fairly rigid. It is also important to remember that Vila-Rovira has a team that allows him to perform the surgery efficiently and with a very well-defined system of fluid replacement, which allows him to perform the procedure with as little risk as possible.

doi:10.1016/j.cps.2007.10.016
plasticsurgery.theclinics.com

ELSEVIER
SAUNDERS

CLINICS IN
PLASTIC
SURGERY

Clin Plastic Surg 35 (2008) 107–114

Upper Body Lift

Shehab Soliman, MD[a], Silvia Cristina Rotemberg, MD[b],
Daniele Pace, MD[c], Adel Bark, MD[c], Alexander Mansur, MD[c],
Albert Cram, MD, FACS[c], Al Aly, MD, FACS[c],*

- Preoperative evaluation
- Operative technique
  Markings
  Positioning

- *Surgical technique*
- Complications
- Summary
- References

The thoracic deformities that develop after massive weight loss are fairly complex. As with any plastic surgery problem, it behooves the plastic surgeon to appropriately define and diagnose the deformity, develop an appreciation of the normal shape that is to be attained in reconstructing it, and then devise a plan to reach that normal shape. Normally, the skin–fat envelope adheres tightly to the underlying musculoskeletal anatomy of the thorax (upper trunk). The inframammary crease has a semicircular shape, with its lateral aspect rising superiorly as the lateral chest wall is approached [1–3].

Weight gain causes the thorax, from the clavicle to the inframammary crease, to expand in a circumferential and a vertical fashion. After weight loss, the thorax deflates in the same way as the cloth covering of a lamp shade would loosen and sag, resulting in two-dimensional excess—circumferential (horizontal) excess and vertical excess (Fig. 1). In the analogy, the inferior edge of the lamp shade expands and lies on the surface on which the lamp sits.

Unlike the lamp shade, the human body has fascial attachments, called zones of adherence, located at the anterior and posterior midlines. The anterior attachment is over the sternum and the posterior attachment is over the spine. During the process of weight gain, the zones of adherence prohibit fat deposition between the skin and the bony anatomy, acting to tether the overlying skin in place. As the patient loses weight, the zones of adherence act as suspension hooks for the hanging thoracic tissues leading to the final configuration of tissues (Box 1).

Thoracic tissues located laterally tend to descend in massive weight loss patients because they are located at the greatest distance from either of the anterior and posterior zones of adherence. The degree to which any of these deformities occurs varies from patient to patient depending on their body mass index, their fat deposition/loss pattern, and the quality of their skin–fat envelope.

Our criteria for operating on patients with upper truncal deformities are similar to those for other regions of the body. The patient has to have stabilized his or her weight loss for at least 3 to 6 months. The key in deciding which procedure or procedures to perform in the upper truncal region is the position of the lateral inframammary crease. If it has "dropped out" or descended, then, by definition, the patient will have upper-back excess in varying degrees and, thus, an upper body lift, in one of its forms, is needed. The authors have performed three forms of upper body lifts (Box 2).

Males are amenable to a full upper body lift, which this article describes. The upper body lift in

[a] Department of Surgery, Cairo University, Kasr El-Aini Hospitals, Cairo, Egypt
[b] Department of Plastic Surgery, Cleveland Clinic, 9500 Euclid Avenue, Cleveland, OH 44195, USA
[c] Iowa City Plastic Surgery, 501 12th Avenue, Suite 102, Coralville, IA 52241
* Corresponding author.
E-mail address: mdplastic@aol.com (A. Aly).

0094-1298/08/$ – see front matter © 2008 Elsevier Inc. All rights reserved.
plasticsurgery.theclinics.com

doi:10.1016/j.cps.2007.09.006

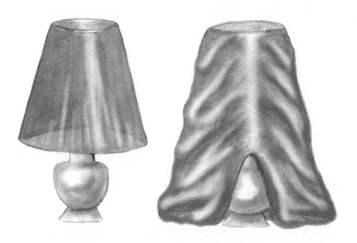

Fig. 1. The lamp shade analogy is helpful in demonstrating how the thoracic region presents in the massive weight loss patient. Like the lamp shade on the right, the thoracic soft tissue drapes toward the table and is held in place by the zones of adherence located in the anterior and posterior midlines. (*From* Aly AS. Upper body lift. In: Aly AS, editor. Body contouring after massive weight loss. St. Louis (MO): Quality Medical Publishing; 2005. p. 337; with permission.)

the male pattern is almost always accompanied by brachioplasty. The lateral thoracic component of the brachioplasty is extended inferiorly to allow for reduction of the horizontal excess that all of these patients present. The upper body lift pattern used to treat females with lateral descent of the inframammary crease depends on the extent of upper-back excess. The article describes both techniques.

If a massive weight loss patient has a normal upward sweeping lateral inframammary crease, he or she presents with upper-arm and breast deformities that are separate from each other and can be treated as such by independent brachioplasty and breast reconstruction procedures. By definition, if the lateral inframammary crease is correctly positioned, the patient does not have upper-back excess and thus does not need to have the thorax treated as a unit.

Preoperative evaluation

The entire thoracic region of a massive weight loss patient is assessed as part of a total body examination. The thickness of the underlying fat is assessed in the anterior, lateral, and posterior regions of the chest. The location and the direction of the lateral inframammary crease in both women and men are assessed. As already mentioned, the key factor in determining whether an upper body lift is to be used in its entirety is the position of the lateral inframammary crease. If it is properly positioned, isolated procedures, such as brachioplasty and breast reshaping surgeries, can be performed. If the lateral crease position is lower than it should be, an upper body lift is appropriate.

Next, the examiner notes the presence or absence of lateral breast rolls, which often continue posteriorly as upper-back rolls. In cases where the lateral inframammary crease is inferiorly displaced, lateral chest tissue should be pinched superiorly to determine the extent of the descent and the amount of improvement in the thoracic contour that could be attained after surgical correction. Continuation of this pinch posteriorly along the path of the upper-back roll also demonstrates the anticipated possible improvement of back contour. A vertical pinch of the posterior axillary fold, which is the extension of upper-arm excess, determines the extent of horizontal thoracic excess.

A massive weight loss patient usually has many areas of complaint, including the thoracic region. The patient and surgeon need to outline all the areas to be addressed and formulate a plan and a schedule for treating different aspects of these deformities. A careful history of weight gain and weight loss should be taken to make sure of weight stability. It is important to make the patient an informed partner in the decision-making process by explaining the extent of deformities, how they

---

Box 1:   Potential thoracic deformities created by massive weight loss

- Anterior and posterior inverted-V deformities
- Lateral inframammary crease descent
- Upper-back excess of varying degrees
- Lateral breast, upper-back rolls
- Breast abnormalities of varying types

    Females: hypertrophy, ptosis, atrophy and ptosis
    Males: variable degrees of gynecomastia

Box 2:   Three patterns for upper body lifts

- Male pattern
- Female pattern type I: for patients with extensive upper-back excess
- Female pattern type II: for patients with mild upper-back excess

were formed, and how they can be treated. Details of the size and scar position are also discussed with the patient. For females, the desired breast size and shape are also discussed so that the appropriate technique to meet these goals is determined. It is often helpful to show photographs of previous surgical results to ensure that the patient has realistic expectations of what can be accomplished.

Operative technique

Markings

The meticulous and precise marking based on the surgical plan is the cornerstone of a successful outcome. It is preferred to do the marking 1 day before surgery. This affords time to adequately photograph the markings, evaluate them, and adjust them before surgery, if needed. Because patients present with varying degrees of deformity, it is important to digest the principles underlying the marking process. Equipped with this knowledge, each surgeon can create his or her marking sequence.

Both the anterior and posterior midlines are marked as reference lines. The patient's natural inframammary crease, which is displaced inferiorly as it traverses laterally, is also marked. The upper arm is marked for brachioplasty using the two-ellipse technique described in the brachioplasty article by Aly and colleagues in this issue. At the lateral edge of the breast, or the lateral part of the inframammary crease, tissues are pinched in a vertical fashion to demonstrate the level where the lateral inframammary crease should be. The full extent of the lateral breast and upper-back rolls is marked using the pinch technique along relaxed skin-tension lines. In some patients, the final resection may reach the posterior midline, while in others, it may not. In male patients, the extension of the brachioplasty over the lateral chest wall extends inferiorly to intersect with the excision of the lateral breast and upper-back rolls, forming an L shape. In most female patients, the two excisions are contiguous but separate. Crosshatch marks are made across the proposed back excision to promote alignment at closure (Fig. 2).

The natural meridian of both breasts is marked in both males and females for orientation during the procedure. Markings are made according to the procedure planned for reconstructing the breast. For men, breast reduction is performed. For women, some need a reduction, others benefit from an augmentation/mastopexy, and still others may only need elevation of the lateral inframammary crease.

Positioning

In the operating room, the patient is first placed in either lateral decubitus position to accommodate

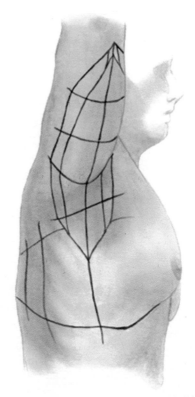

Fig. 2. Marking for a male-type upper body lift. (*From* Aly AS. Upper body lift. In: Aly AS, editor. Body contouring after massive weight loss. St. Louis (MO): Quality Medical Publishing; 2005. p. 345; with permission.)

the brachioplasty and the excisions of the lateral breast and upper-back rolls on one side. The patient is then turned to the other lateral decubitus position to accommodate the same procedure on the opposite side. Finally, the patient is put in the supine position to permit operation on the breasts.

Surgical technique

Male pattern

After induction of general anesthesia, the patient is placed in the lateral decubitus position. An axillary roll is used and all pressure points are padded. The operating team of surgeons needs 360° access to operate on both the arm and upper back. This can be accomplished by turning the head of the table 180° from the anesthesiologist or by moving the table far enough away from the anesthesia equipment to allow access. The patient is then prepped and draped. The brachioplasty procedure is performed first. In male cases, the lateral chest wall component of the brachioplasty is closed with temporary staples to allow for adjustments during the breast component of the procedure. (In female cases, the

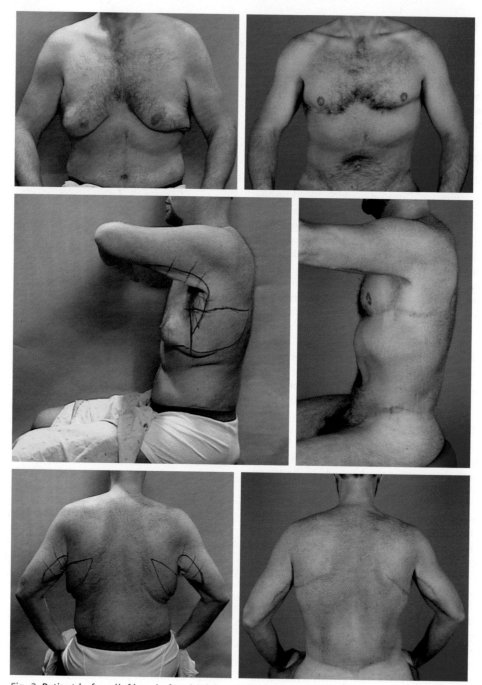

Fig. 3. Patient before (*left*) and after (*right*) a male-pattern upper body lift.

procedure is performed as described in the brachio-plasty article by Aly and colleagues in this issue.)

After the brachioplasty component is accom-plished, the proposed superior extent of the lateral breast and upper-back rolls is incised down to the level of the underlying muscle fascia. An inferiorly based skin–fat flap is elevated down to the pro-posed inferior level of resection. Next, with the

flap elevated superiorly while the shoulder is pushed inferiorly, the flap is tailored to the superior line of excision. Closure is accomplished in two layers with an overlying layer of skin glue. A closed suction is placed in the area of resection.

At this point of the procedure, upper-arm excess is eliminated, the lateral breast and upper-back rolls are eliminated, the lateral inframammary crease is

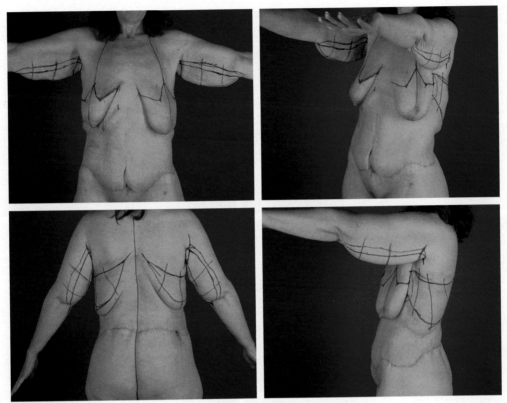

Fig. 4. Typical marking for a female type I pattern upper body lift.

elevated to its proper position, and a "dog ear" is created at the lateral inferior pole of the breast, especially in male patients.

After both sides are completed, the patient is placed in the supine position to perform the planned breast reconstruction.

In men, a gynecomastia procedure is planned. For women, the plan varies according to the deformity and the patient's desires. In the gynecomastia procedure, the inframammary crease, in its elevated proper lateral position, is incised and the dissection is taken down to the level of the underlying muscle fascia. This maneuver usually results in the crease falling down and away from its original position because of gravity and lack of good adherence of the inframammary crease in the massive weight loss patient. To reconstruct the crease in its superior position, it is sutured with large permanent sutures to the underlying rib perichondrium at the appropriate level along the entire length of the crease. In some patients, this is fairly close to the inferior border of the pectoralis muscle. In others, it is slightly lower.

Superiorly the breast tissue is elevated at the level of the pectoralis fascia up to the second rib. The nipple–areolar complex is harvested as a full thickness graft with an approximate diameter of 2.5 cm in males. The temporary staples from the lateral chest wall closure of the brachioplasty are removed and the breast flap is advanced inferiorly and laterally in a "vest over pants" manner. The excess is tailored inferiorly and laterally. A closed suction drain is placed in the breast pocket through separate incisions, and the wound is closed in layers. After checking both breasts for symmetry, the new positions for the nipple–areola complexes are marked. The authors feel that the best position for the nipple–areolar complex in a male is just lateral to the meridian and slightly above the inframammary crease. A 2.5-cm circular area is de-epithelized where the nipple–areolar complex is to be placed and the full thickness graft is applied.

Fig. 3 shows a patient before and 1 year after an upper body lift. Note the elimination of the anterior and posterior inverted "V" deformities; elevation of the entire inframammary crease, especially its lateral component; and the elimination of the upper-back roll. By leaving some excess fat on the tailored breast flap, it is possible to give the impression that the patient has some fullness to his pectoralis muscle, which can be aesthetically pleasing.

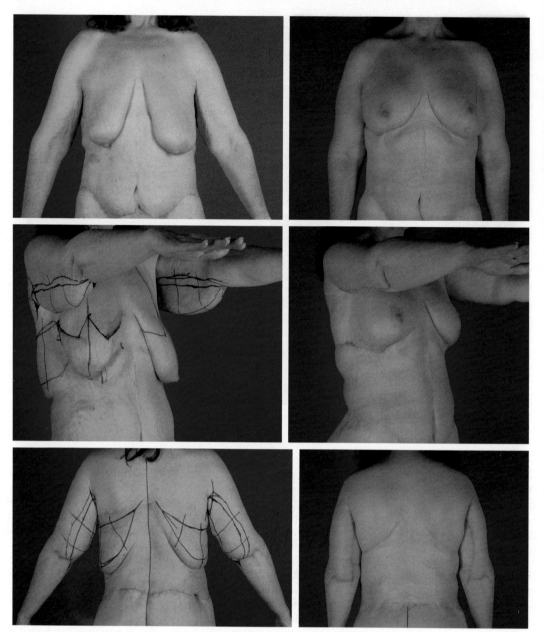

Fig. 5. Patient before (*left*) and after (*right*) undergoing an upper body lift using a female type I pattern of resection.

Female pattern type I and type II

In most female massive weight loss patients that have a "dropped out" lateral inframammary crease, an upper body lift is required to eliminate upper-back excess. The upper-back excess can present in a variety of forms anywhere from extensive upper-back rolls to mild excess. The upper body lift also lifts the lateral inframammary crease to its appropriate position to create an appropriate base upon which the breast can be reconstructed. In the male-patient pattern described above, the lateral

thoracic excision of the brachioplasty component of an upper body lift is very aggressive to eliminate the horizontal thoracic excess. In females, horizontal excess does not necessarily need to be eliminated because the accompanying breast reconstruction usually requires some horizontal excess to accommodate the increased projection. Thus, in many patients, the pattern of excision from the brachioplasty component does not connect with the excision of the upper-back and lateral breast rolls (Fig. 4).

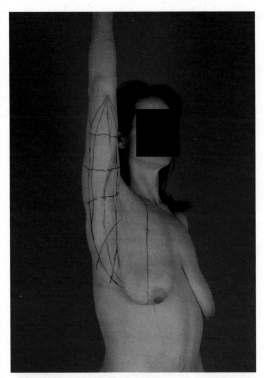

Fig. 6. Patient marked for an upper body lift using female type II pattern.

We call this female pattern type I and it is the most common pattern used in females in our practice. Ideal patients for this procedure have a large amount of upper-back excess, which requires a bra-line excision to create the appropriate contour. Another important consideration in the female patient is that in creating the lines of excision, the lateral border of the breast has to be respected. Thus, it must be left intact. As in the male pattern of upper body lifting, the inframammary crease usually requires reinforcement by attaching it to its proper position with deep permanent utures that go through the underlying rib perichondrium. Fig. 5 shows a woman after undergoing an upper body lift using female pattern type I. Note the lateral inframammary crease elevation, elimination of upper-back excess, and the improvement in arm contour.

Females who present with a minimal amount of upper-back excess that only manifests itself as loose tissue apparent above a worn bra are good candidates for female pattern type II upper body lifts. This pattern eliminates the excess through a continuation of the brachioplasty excision down through the lateral chest to the inframammary crease (Fig. 6).

Because the upper-back excess is minimal, the excisional pattern allows for the upward rotation of upper-back tissue along the entire length of the excision. This, as with all upper body lift techniques, elevates the lateral inframammary crease to its proper position (Fig. 7).

With this pattern of excision, the surgeon must be careful not to lateralize the breast. Thus, to prevent breast lateralization, it may be warranted to perform the breast procedure first when using this pattern so that the resection can be adjusted.

Complications

Outside of complications of bleeding, infection, and potential unattractive scarring, which are common to all surgical procedures, the most common complications of upper body lifts are wound separation and/or dehiscence, usually occurring near the lateral aspect of the breast. These are probably due to the significant tension created at this point and the strain that simple turning movements of the trunk can put on closure in this region. Resecting less tissue in this area may reduce the likelihood of problems. However, that choice has to be weighed against under-resection, which can lead to persistent fullness in the upper-back region.

Seromas can occur in the upper-back component or in the breast region. They are treated by serial aspirations and tend to resolve without surgical intervention. Another problem that can be encountered is a loose inframammary crease, which may not support large implants should they need to be used in the breast reconstruction. This can lead to the implant falling through the crease. To prevent this problem, the inframammary crease should be supported by suturing the deep tissues to the appropriate underlying rib perichondrium.

The complications associated with the brachioplasty component of an upper body lift are the same as those encountered with brachioplasty and are discussed in the brachioplasty article by Aly and colleagues in this issue.

Summary

An upper body lift is needed whenever a massive weight loss patient presents with a "dropped out" lateral inframammary crease. It is a combination of a brachioplasty, upper-back resection, and breast reconstruction. The operation is designed to reverse the particular deformity a patient presents. This article described three patterns of resection, one for males and two for females.

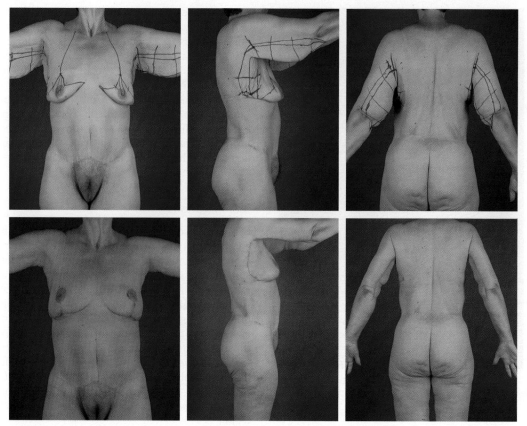

Fig. 7. Patient who underwent an upper body lift using female type II pattern. Before (*top row*). After (*bottom row*).

References

[1] Aly AS. Upper body lift. In: Aly AS, editor. Body contouring after massive weight loss. St. Louis (MO): Quality Medical Publishing; 2005. p. 335–60.

[2] Aly A, Cram AE, Pace D. Brachioplasty in the patient with massive weight loss. Aesthetic Surg J 2006;26:76–84.

[3] Aly AS, Cram AE. Brachioplasty. In: Aly AS, editor. Body contouring after massive weight loss. St. Louis (MO): Quality Medical Publishing; 2005. p. 303–33.

ELSEVIER
SAUNDERS

CLINICS IN
PLASTIC
SURGERY

Clin Plastic Surg 35 (2008) 115–120

Lateral Thoracic Excisions in the Post Massive Weight Loss Patient

Susan E. Downey, MD, FACS*, John E. Gross, MD

As the field of postbariatric plastic surgery increases, more patients are seen with excess skin and fat in areas of the body not previously considered. The traditional techniques do not always achieve the desired results. New techniques need to be developed to expand on the traditional techniques and to address surrounding areas. New techniques, such as the vertical thoracic resection, often develop when patients have been treated with traditional methods but then come in and request that additional adjacent areas be treated.

Redundant skin and fat can be seen anywhere on the body following massive weight loss. The lateral chest can have an excess of skin and fat as well as anywhere else on the body. The lateral chest area is particularly troublesome in light of current female fashions. Many women's fashions include T-shirts or other tops made out of clingy fabrics, not the looser, less shape-defining blouses of the past. In many women, wearing a bra makes the redundancy most evident, with the excess skin and fat bulging over the top. Traditional techniques of brachioplasty, with the scar ending in the axilla, as well as the traditional techniques of mastopexy, with the inframammary scar ending no further than the lateral extent of the breast, do not address this excess. Fig. 1 shows a patient who underwent a traditional brachioplasty, with the scar ending in the axilla, as well as a traditional mastopexy, with the scar ending at the lateral edge of the breast. She presented with the complaint of persistent lateral chest wall fullness. This excess was magnified and clearly visible when she was wearing a bra. A technique was used to extend the brachioplasty excision laterally down the chest wall to maximally remove the excess skin and fat; the scar was placed in an area hidden under the arm while it is at rest along the lateral thorax (Figs. 2–5). Most of the lateral chest excess can be addressed by an incision extending from the axilla to the inframammary fold. This can be done independently or as part of a brachioplasty. At the time of assessment for a brachioplasty, it can be determined if lateral chest excess exists; if so, an extended brachioplasty can be configured that will include lateral chest wall excision (Fig. 6). If a patient has had a previous traditional brachioplasty, the lateral chest wall excision can be performed separately.

The lateral excision can be extended down the entire length of the body (Fig. 7). Following massive weight gain and then loss, there are vertical and horizontal excesses of remaining skin and fat. Lower abdominal incisions for an abdominoplasty/panniculectomy or even for a more extensive lower body lift/belt lipectomy do not address horizontal excess of the abdominal wall. In patients who have a midline incision, this incision has been used to remove additional excess skin and fat in the horizontal direction. As the popularity of laparoscopic procedures increases, the incidence of preexisting midline incisions decreases; however, patients may still want to address the residual laxity

Keck School of Medicine, University of Southern California, Los Angeles, CA, USA
* Corresponding author. 1301 Twentieth Street, Suite 470, Santa Monica, CA 90404.
E-mail address: sdowneymd@aol.com (S.E. Downey).

doi:10.1016/j.cps.2007.08.003

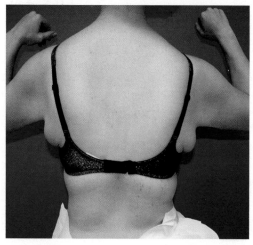

Fig. 1. Patient with lateral chest fullness following massive weight loss.

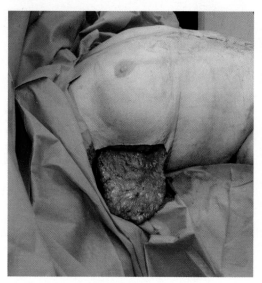

Fig. 3. Excision of lateral chest wall fullness.

of the back and the anterior abdomen. For this patient, an extension of the lateral thoracic incision along the lateral abdominal wall can address the abdominal excess as well as back laxity. Although the patient will have a long scar laterally, this may be more desirable than a midline incision for some patients. The first stage is the lower abdominal incision; however, for the patient complaining of residual horizontal anterior abdominal excess or residual back excess, a lateral thoracic excision might be appropriate at a later time.

Potential complications of seroma and skin loss can occur with any procedure after massive weight loss. This approach is not immune to these

problems. Because this technique does not include undermining and basically is a wedge excision of loose tissue, the risk for skin loss is minimal, even in patients who previously have undergone a lower body lift. Seromas can occur, and the use of drains is recommended.

The markings for the excision must be done in the standing upright position. The tissues are pinched, and the excess is determined. Markings are done for the proposed wedge excision, and these are followed on the operating table. As the tissue falls away when the patient is placed on the operating table, preoperative markings are critical. Hash marks can be used to realign the tissues and are particularly helpful when an upward pull is desired to correct a downward sloping inframammary fold. When a lateral chest wall excision is planned at the same time as a brachioplasty, it is useful to mark the inframammary fold as the lowest point of the proposed incision, as well as the lateral extent of the breast. An easy way to mark is to push all of the lax tissue anteriorly, mark a vertical line that will be the desired point of the final incision, and then fold back the lax tissue and mark the extent of the excision. This method allows for the resulting scar to be well hidden under the arm when it is at rest. Asymmetries may exist as in so many other procedures, and these are evaluated best in the standing erect position. As a general rule, these excisions should not be made at the same time as a lower abdominal incision (eg, abdominoplasty or lower body lift), but should be done a minimum of 3 months later to allow the blood supply to develop to the previously elevated abdominal flaps.

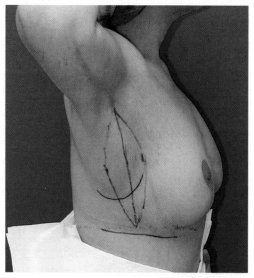

Fig. 2. Markings for proposed excision of lateral chest fullness.

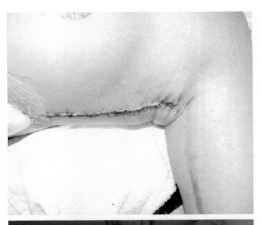

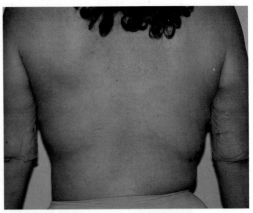

Fig. 5. Posterior view after excision of lateral chest excess.

Dr Aly makes the analogy of the upper body after weight loss being like a curtain. The analogy describes the obese thoracic soft tissues that are deflated by massive weight loss. After massive weight loss, the tissues hang lower on the underlying skeleton than previously, except at the zones of adherence located at the anterior and posterior midlines. Even during massive weight gain fat does not increase under these zones of adherence. Dr Aly's curtain analogy describes loose deflated tissues draping down from a central tethering point, much like draperies hanging down from a central secure point. The fascial attachments lead to

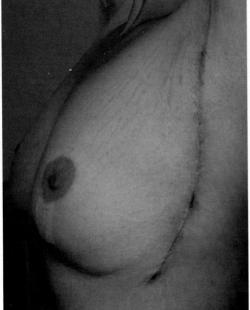

Fig. 4. Closure after excision of lateral chest wall fullness.

Aly [1] described the descent of tissues after massive weight loss. This descent is not uniform and is subject to zones of adherence. To define the goals of surgery after massive weight loss, one must understand the normal. The goal is to restore the body to as close to normal as possible. The normal upper trunk has a skin–fat envelope that is tightly adherent to the underlying musculoskeletal anatomy. The normal inframammary crease has a semicircular shape, with its lateral aspect rising superiorly as the lateral chest wall is approached. As the body loses large amounts of excess weight, there is a residual excess in the vertical and horizontal dimensions. Fascial attachments are located at the anterior (sternum) and posterior (spine) midlines, with the excess skin and residual fat draping off these attachments and sweeping down laterally and inferiorly.

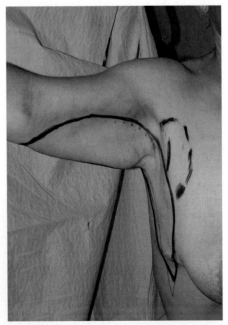

Fig. 6. Markings for excision of lateral chest wall fullness at same time as brachioplasty.

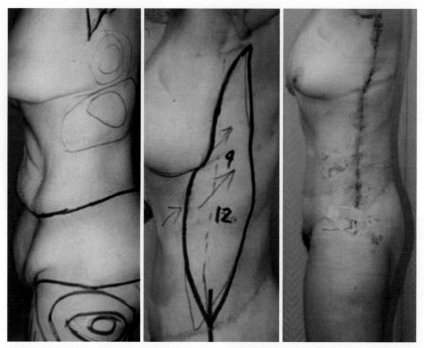

Fig. 7. Markings for vertical thoracic excision. (*From* Rahban SR, Gross JE. A new approach to correction of truncal redundancy after massive weight loss–the lateral thoracoabdominoplasty. Aesthetic Surg J 2007;27:518–523; with permission. Copyright © 2007 by The American Society for Aesthetic Plastic Surgery, Inc.)

inverted-V deformities of the breast tissue inferiorly and the upper back posteriorly. The lateral aspect of the inframammary crease descends as it traverses from medial to lateral, because the lateral thoracic tissues are located at the greatest distance from either of the adherent fascial attachments. Thus, the patient has vertical excess, most dramatically manifested in the descent of the lateral inframammary crease, and horizontal excess around the circumference of the thorax [1].

The lateral descent of the breast and the inframammary fold can be telling stigmata of massive weight loss. Breast surgery, such as mastopexy, alone does not address this issue. A lateral chest wall excision can elevate the inframammary fold and reposition the lateral aspect of the breast. With this correction of the inframammary fold, the breast may appear rejuvenated without any direct surgical intervention (Fig. 8).

An interesting adjunct to the lateral thoracic excision has been the use of this excess tissue to autoaugment the breast. Patients who have lost massive amounts of excess weight often present with deflated breasts. Because of the blood supplies that had developed during their weight gain and the laxity of the tissues, mobilization of lateral chest wall excess can be done to a degree that is not possible in patients who have not experienced the extremes of weight gain and loss. Mobilization of this tissue and rotation of the tissue under the breast can be used for a modest autoaugmentation. For some patients, this might be an adequate augmentation and may be preferable to a prosthetic augmentation.

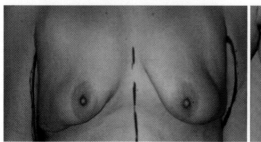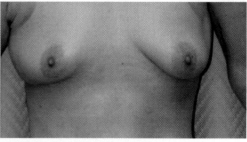

Fig. 8. Lateral descent of inframammary fold and correction by lateral thoracic excision only.

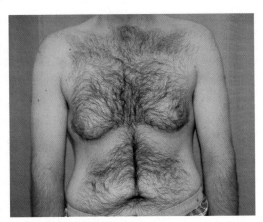

Fig. 9. Preoperative gynecomastia.

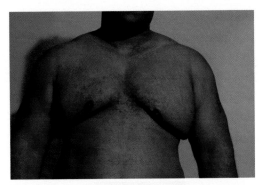

Fig. 11. Male chest after massive weight loss.

As in so many other areas of plastic surgery, the male patient offers many anatomic problems that are different from those seen in the female patient. The chest area often is of concern to the male patient who has lost a massive amount of weight, and it may be the first area that he wishes to address with plastic surgery. Many male patients are concerned about visible scars although they wish an extensive removal of skin and fat. One of the many ways in which men differ from women is in the public baring of their chests. With few exceptions, women do not bare their chests in public; therefore, even with skimpy bathing costumes there are opportunities for the plastic surgeon to hide scars. Conversely, men remove or wish to remove their shirts frequently in public, while sitting by the pool, while on the beach, when playing sports (shirts on one team and bare chests on the other for basketball pick-up games), or even when mowing the lawn. Therefore, different surgical methods need to be used for the male chest. Just to reduce the volume and leave the patient with visible scars, which continue to inhibit the man from

participating fully in social and sporting events, does not accomplish the goals of the surgery.

The treatment of gynecomastia has evolved for all patients from the previously used methods with large excisions of skin and fat to newer methods of minimal scar approaches. Hammond and colleagues [2] described a method with the only scar being one in the anterior axillary line. Through this incision, ultrasonic liposuction of the entire chest area, as well as direct excision of fibrous breast tissue, can be done. We have found this technique to be readily adaptable to the chest of the man who has lost a massive amount of weight. An observation has been that the skin of the male chest shows excellent contraction and appears to contract better than skin elsewhere (Figs. 9 and 10).

One successful approach has been to combine lateral excisions with extensive liposuction of the chest area. This may require a two-stage approach. Liposuction and even direct excision may be necessary to reduce significant gynecomastia. Direct excision of breast tissue and liposuction can be accomplished through the small incision in the anterior axillary line, as described by Hammond and colleagues. Liposuction also can be done of the lateral folds to deflate this area. In general, we have found that ultrasonic liposuction is more useful in reducing the male chest than is traditional

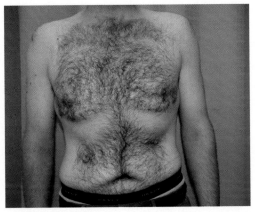

Fig. 10. Postoperative gynecomastia after use of pull-through technique.

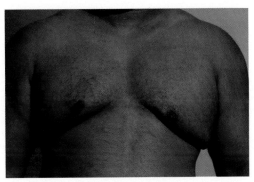

Fig. 12. Male chest after first-stage liposuction.

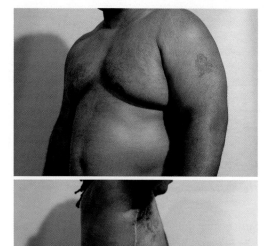

Fig. 13. Male chest after second-stage lateral thoracic excision.

liposuction. When liposuction is done as a first stage to reduce lateral folds, a waiting period of at least 3 months is necessary to allow the swelling to go down. At that time, an excision of the lateral chest can be accomplished. The incision will extend from the axilla to the inferior border of the pectoralis (Figs. 11–13). This scar is well hidden when the arms are by the side and is tolerated well, even by athletic men.

The lateral vertical thoracic excision has been a useful adjunct to more traditional techniques. As more patients undergo massive weight loss, more patients will present to plastic surgeons with complaints of fullness and excess in areas of the body not addressed by more traditional techniques. The lateral vertical thoracic excision can offer a solution to a difficult problem.

References

[1] Aly AS. Body contouring after massive weight loss. St. Louis: Quality Medical Publishing; 2006.

[2] Hammond DC, Arnold JF, Simon AM, et al. Combined use of ultrasonic liposuction with the pull through technique for treatment of gynecomastia. Plast Reconstr Surg 2003;112(3):891–5; discussion 896–7.

ELSEVIER
SAUNDERS

CLINICS IN
PLASTIC
SURGERY

Clin Plastic Surg 35 (2008) 121

Editorial Commentary

The thoracic or upper truncal region in many patients who have undergone massive weight loss is distorted by weight gain and weight loss. Often patients concentrate their complaints around the breast area, whether male or female. If probed, however, many are unhappy with their entire thoracic region, which includes the breast, lateral thorax, and upper back regions. Patients most often use terminology such as "I hate this roll above my bra," or "I want to get rid of this roll that did not go away after my body lift." It thus behooves the plastic surgeon to develop strategies to address this entire area. The two preceding articles address the thoracic region as a unit in dramatically different ways. What they share, however, is more important. They both address lateral inframammary crease descent, which is synonymous with upper back excess.

0094-1298/08/$ – see front matter © 2008 Elsevier Inc. All rights reserved.
plasticsurgery.theclinics.com

doi:10.1016/j.cps.2007.10.017

ELSEVIER
SAUNDERS

CLINICS IN
PLASTIC
SURGERY

Clin Plastic Surg 35 (2008) 123–129

Mastopexy After Massive Weight Loss: Dermal Suspension and Selective Auto-Augmentation

J. Peter Rubin, MD*, Gerald Khachi, MD

- The nature of breast deformities after weight loss
- Patient evaluation
- Choice of technique
- Authors' technique
- Discussion
- Summary
- References

Since ancient times, the female breast has been portrayed by artists on canvas and sculptures. This breadth of artistic rendering spans from the Paleolithic Period with Venus of Willendorf, 24,000 BC, to the more recent abstract paintings of Willem de-Kooning. Despite changes in ideal concepts of beauty throughout the ages, a common thread is found among these images. The female breast has been depicted consistently as nonptotic, evenly contoured, and youthful. This image of youthfulness is equated with health and beauty in modern society. Patients who successfully undergo massive weight loss desire to shed the physical signs of a formerly obese person and adopt a renewed body image. Many patients are troubled by the breast deformities following weight loss and find that mastopexy has a positive impact on their body image. We describe a technique, which uses principles of dermal suspension and parenchymal reshaping, that allows for selective auto-augmentation of the breast with lateral chest wall tissue.

The nature of breast deformities after weight loss

The youthful breast is located between the second and fifth intercostal space. The inferior mammary fold (IMF) is located below the nipple areolar complex (NAC). The IMF to nipple distance is 6 to 8 cm. The sternal notch to nipple distance usually measures 19 to 21 cm in a youthful breast. NAC represents the point of maximum projection on the breast at the midclavicular line.

Ptosis refers to inferior and lateral descent of the NAC in relation to the IMF and breast parenchyma, and a common classification system defines first-degree or mild ptosis as a nipple position within 1 cm of the IMF. In second-degree, or moderate, ptosis, the nipple is 1 to 3 cm below the IMF and on the anterior projection of the breast mound. In third-degree, major ptosis, the NAC is below the IMF and on the dependent portion of the inferior breast pole [1]. This classification system, however, falls short of defining the breast deformities that are seen after massive weight loss. Massive weight loss results in severe breast volume deflation with flattening and inelastic skin that deforms and distorts breast tissue. Additionally, nipple position becomes more medialized, and axillary skin rolls blur the borders between the lateral breast and chest wall. In the face of these changes, traditional mastopexy techniques are inadequate [2].

University of Pittsburgh, Plastic and Reconstructive Surgery, Scaife Hall, Suite 682, 3550 Terrace Street, Pittsburgh, PA 15261, USA
* Corresponding author.
E-mail address: rubinjp@upmc.edu (J.P. Rubin).

doi:10.1016/j.cps.2007.08.008

Patient evaluation

Management of breast ptosis in patients with significant weight loss, as is seen in the gastric bypass population, can be challenging. The desired goals and expectations of the patient must be investigated. Unrealistic goals and preconceived ideals need to be addressed before surgery. During the same consultation, a full history and focused physical examination are performed. We require mammographic imaging consistent with the screening guidelines of the American Cancer

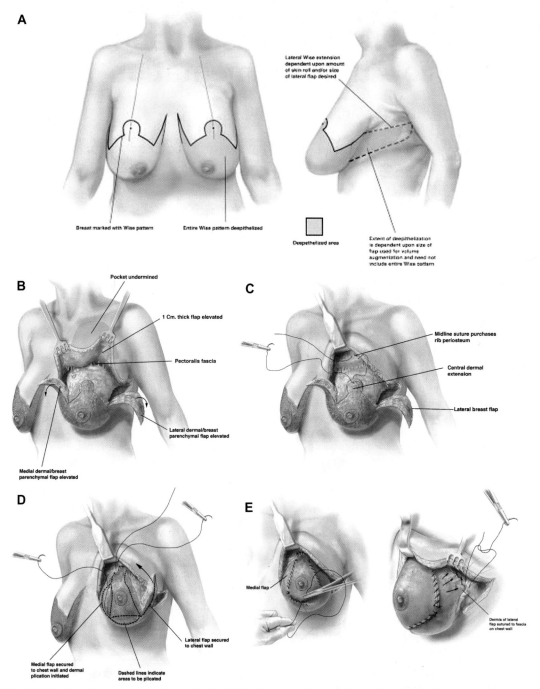

Fig. 1. (*A–F*) Operative sequence. (*From* Rubin, JP. Mastopexy in the massive weight loss patient: dermal suspension and total parenchymal reshaping. Aesthetic Surgery Journal 2006;26:214–22; with permission. Copyright © 2006 by The American Society for Aesthetic Plastic Surgery, Inc.)

F

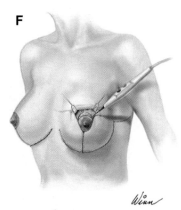

Wénn

Fig. 1 (continued)

Choice of technique

For patients with only mild deformities, many standard techniques can be used. A comprehensive review of the types of mastopexy is beyond the scope of this article; however, the following simple algorithm may be followed. Those who have mild ptosis and are content with their breast size may need only mastopexy with periareolar skin reduction [4]. Moderate ptosis and skin laxity require the NAC to be moved more superiorly, with excision of vertical skin from the NAC down to the IMF [5,6]. Severe ptosis requires an additional horizontal excision at the IMF, resulting in an inverted T incision.

Patients with mild ptosis and who are unsatisfied with their breast size require alloplastic augmentation, and this alone may correct the ptosis. Those with moderate to severe ptosis in addition to unacceptable breast volume also require augmentation with mastopexy. Consideration should be given to staging these procedures. Caution should be exercised when treating patients with previous breast augmentation presenting with ptosis. Explantation in conjunction with mastopexy and capsulotomy may compromise blood supply to the skin and nipple [7].

For patients with adequate parenchymal volume, but severe ptosis and flattening of the breast shape, we recommend a technique that allows for suspension of the breast tissue to rib periosteum to achieve

Society [3] and basic laboratory studies. The breast deformities should be defined precisely, with attention to laxity of the skin envelope, existing breast parenchymal volume, IMF position, presence of lateral skin roll, potential medial position of the nipple, and asymmetry. Relative contraindications to surgery include previous breast scars, severe fibrocystic disease, active severe intertrigo, and other active dermatologic conditions. We routinely exclude tobacco users. Consideration should be given to how the mastopexy procedure will fit into an operative plan involving multiple concurrent procedures or staged procedures.

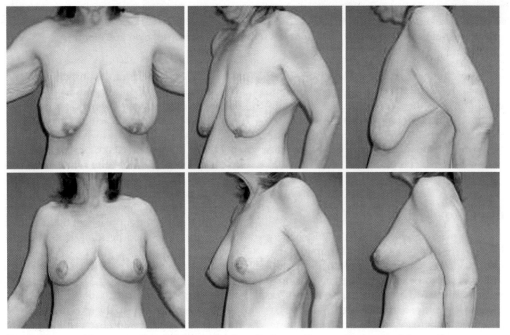

Fig. 2. 46-year-old woman after 160-lb weight loss. Postoperative results shown at 6 months.

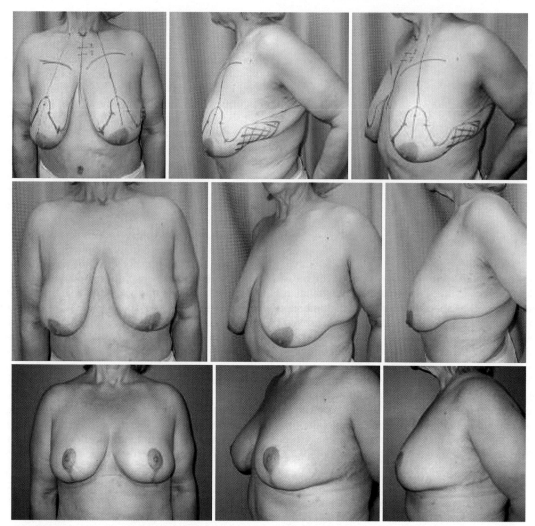

Fig. 3. 42-year-old woman after 140-lb weight loss. Postoperative results shown at 6 months.

superior pole fullness. A lateral chest wall flap is used to selectively add tissue to the breast mound while eliminating the lateral skin roll deformity [8]. Although this technique does involve more extensive scars compared with other mastopexy techniques, patients who are willing to accept the scars are satisfied with the procedure.

Authors' technique

We base our markings on an extended Wise pattern with preservation of the inferior and central pedicle. Nipple position is marked in relation to the IMF and often needs to be moved more laterally along a symmetrically drawn breast meridian. The vertical limb of the keyhole pattern measures 5 cm. The lateral marking of the Wise pattern is extended posteriorly to encompass the axillary skin roll. This serves

two purposes: it removes the unsightly lateral skin rolls, and it assists in autologous augmentation of the breast parenchyma. Robust perforators in the lateral thoracic region allow this flap to be mobilized. The areola is marked with a 42-mm cookie cutter. The purple shaded area shown in Fig. 1A is de-epithelialized. Of note, the area marked "lateral Wise extension" may be de-epithelialized completely or partially, depending on the amount of tissue needed for auto-augmentation. We recommend de-epithelializing the entire length of the roll, creating the flap, and then deciding if it needs to be trimmed.

The remaining breast parenchyma is degloved by elevating flap that are 1- to 1.5-cm thick (Fig. 1B). Upon reaching the pectoralis major fascia, continue undermining the tissue to the level of the clavicle to create a large pocket. Mobilize the lateral and medial flaps of the breast tissue down to the chest

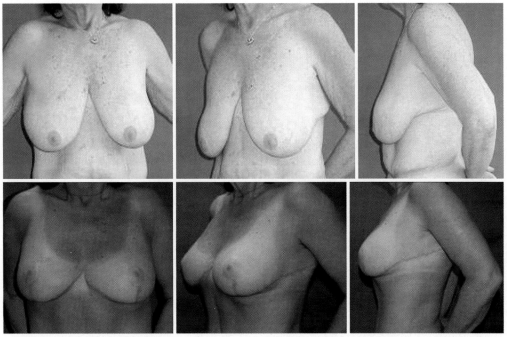

Fig. 4. 57-year-old woman after 130-lb weight loss. Postoperative results shown at 10 months.

wall fascia, taking care to preserve perforators at the base. These are the parts of the Wise pattern that ordinarily would be discarded in a breast reduction. The lateral flap may be extended to the posterior axillary line and beyond to add tissue to the breast. When dealing with an extended flap, check for healthy bleeding at the margin before mobilizing the flap into the breast mound.

Next, suspend the central dermal extension to the rib periosteum as shown in Fig. 1C. Identify the appropriate rib level, and mark the area along the breast meridian. The level is chosen based on the distance between the central dermal extension and the nipple. This usually is the second rib. With the nondominant hand, palpate the intercostal space above and below the selected rib level. Maintaining your fingers in the intercostal space ensures the correct path of the 0-braided suture into periosteum. A few extra moments spent on exposure along with ensuring a good purchase of the periosteum is invaluable. This ultimately places the nipple close to the final position intended. In a similar fashion, the lateral breast flap is secured to the chest wall by way of periosteal tacking sutures. The lateral flap may be sutured at the same or one rib level inferior to the central suspension. The medial flap is secured in a similar fashion. An additional two to three suspension sutures may be used for reinforcement. To shape the dermis, use 2-0 absorbable sutures to plicate the broad surface areas

of the flaps (Fig. 1D). Begin by approximating the lateral dermal flap to the central dermal extension. Next, plicate the medial flap in a similar manner.

To increase nipple projection and shorten NAC to IMF distance, plicate the inferior pole of the breast. This distance is set at 5 cm (Fig. 1E).

To ensure symmetry, it is advantageous to perform each suspension and plication simultaneously on both breasts, rather than completing one and performing the second based on recall. Additionally, the suspension and shaping is done with the patient in a sitting position. We have found that the pattern of plication is tailored to each patient. Thus, placement of additional plication sutures to attain the desired shape may be necessary.

Next, the edge of the lateral dermal flap is secured to the chest wall fascia (Fig. 1E). It is not necessary to secure this to the periosteum, but simply the fascia. This prevents lateral bulging and enhances nipple projection. This maneuver defines the lateral curvature of the breast. Constant redraping of the skin flap assists with any minor adjustments. Finally, skin closure is performed with buried interrupted and running absorbable sutures in the dermis. During closure, the nipple may be tethered or malpositioned. Using cautery, release the tethered dermis to allow the nipple to sit at the desired location (Fig. 1F). It is safe to release the dermis more than halfway around the circumference of the areola, given the robust central pedicle blood

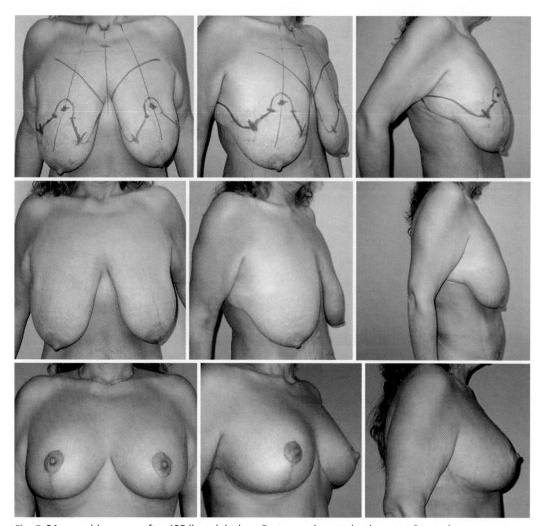

Fig. 5. 34-year-old woman after 135-lb weight loss. Postoperative results shown at 3 months.

supply. Nipple closure is performed with intradermal sutures, and suction drains are placed in each lateral breast.

Representative clinical cases are shown in Figs. 2–6.

Discussion

Morbid obesity in the United States has reached startling proportions. It is estimated that 144,000 gastric bypasses were performed in 2004 [9]. As the number of bariatric cases increase, there will be an equally increasing demand for body contouring after weight loss. The actual weight loss and the body-contouring surgery after weight loss have beneficial effects on self-esteem and body image [10]. In particular, breast reshaping is a popular focus for the patient who has lost weight.

The breast deformities that are seen in patients with massive weight loss are not addressed with traditional mastopexy techniques. Our approach eliminates the lateral skin rolls, while providing volume augmentation to the breast. Suspension of breast parenchyma to pectoralis fascia has been supported by other investigators [11,12]. Recurrence of ptosis is less likely with suspension to rib periosteum.

Major complications have included one hematoma requiring operative drainage and two cases of wound dehiscence treated with dressing changes until healed. Minor wound dehiscence at the triple point has been observed in 5% of our patients. There have been no cases of nipple loss, major tissue loss, of detectable fat necrosis. Flap viability is confirmed with brisk intraoperative bleeding at the tip. Similar transposition flaps have been used with success in breast surgery [13].

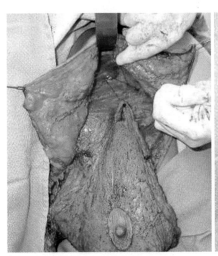
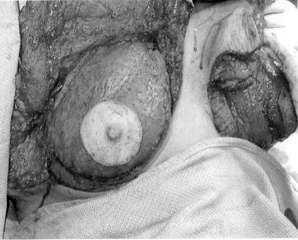

Fig. 6. Intraoperative photographs of patient in *Fig. 5,* demonstrating dermal suspension and breast shape after suspension and placation, but before breast flap is closed. Note that the patient is in a sitting position, and the breast tissue is secured firmly to the chest wall.

Summary

The technique that we outlined is extremely versatile for restoring an esthetic and youthful breast shape in the patient who has lost a massive amount of weight. Overall, complication rates have been low. Despite the disadvantages of a lengthy scar and the need for extensive intraoperative tailoring (which may increase operative time), this operation carries an extremely high rate of patient satisfaction.

References

[1] Regnault P. Breast ptosis: definition and treatment. Clin Plast Surg 1976;3(2):193–203.

[2] Song AY, Jean RD, Hurwitz DJ, et al. A classification of contour deformities after bariatric weight lost: the Pittsburgh rating scale. Plast Reconstr Surg 2005;116(5):1535–44.

[3] American Cancer Society. Detailed guide: breast cancer. 2007. Available at: http://www.cancer.org/docroot/CRI/CRI_2_3x.asp?dt=5. Accessed September 10, 2007.

[4] Benelli L. A new periareolar mammaplasty: the "round block" technique. Aesthetic Plast Surg 1990;14:93–100.

[5] Lassus C. Update on vertical mammaplasty. Plast Reconstr Surg 1999;104:2289–302.

[6] Lejour M. Vertical mammaplasty and liposuction of the breast. St Louis (MO): Quality Medical Publishing; 1993.

[7] Handel N. Secondary mastopexy in the augmented patient: a recipe for disaster. Plast Reconstr Surg 2006;118(7S):152–63.

[8] Rubin JP. Mastopexy in the massive weight loss patient: dermal suspension and total parenchymal reshaping. Aesthetic Surgery Journal 2006; 26:214–22.

[9] Wolfe BL, Terry ML. Expectations and outcomes with gastric bypass surgery. Obes Surg 2006;16: 1622–9.

[10] Song A, Rubin JP, Thomas V, et al. Shifting bodies, shifting ideals: assessment of body image and quality of life in post-bariatric weight loss body contouring patients. Obesity (Silver Spring) 2006;14:1626–36.

[11] Graf R, Biggs T. In search of better shape in mastopexy and reduction mammoplasty. Plast Reconstr Surg 2002;110:309–17.

[12] Frey M. A new technique in mammaplasty: dermis suspension and elimination of medial scars. Br J Plast Surg 1999;52:45–51.

[13] Holmstrom H. The lateral thoracodorsal flap in breast reconstruction. Plast Reconstr Surg 1986; 77:933–43.

CLINICS IN
PLASTIC
SURGERY

Clin Plastic Surg 35 (2008) 131–140

ELSEVIER
SAUNDERS

L Brachioplasty Correction of Excess Tissue of the Upper Arm, Axilla, and Lateral Chest

Dennis J. Hurwitz, MD, FACS[a,b,*], Tim Neavin, MD[c]

- Deformity
- Patient selection and goals
- Operative technique
- The operation

- Discussion
- Summary
- References

The upper arm, axilla, and adjacent chest of a woman are appreciated for femininity, beauty, and erotic sensuality. As such, the excess sagging skin and fat in this area that commonly follows massive weight loss or aging is exceptionally annoying. Although the most dramatic manifestation is the canopy-like draping between the axilla and the elbow, disturbing deformity sometimes extends distally onto the forearm but invariably includes the axilla and crosses onto the chest and lateral breast.

These afflicted women awkwardly cover up with long sleeves. They disdain sleeveless tops and bathing suits. Lateral skin rolls annoyingly overhang the top edge of their bra. Excessively deep and oversized armpits look bizarre and are difficult to shave.

Brachioplasty is the plastic operation that treats this common condition [1–4]. By its most limited definition, brachioplasty removes excess medial upper arm skin and fat for esthetic reshaping. Patients with the moderate to severe deformity have taught us that brachioplasty should be expanded to include the axilla and upper chest. The new contour throughout this region should be attractive, the scars inconspicuous, and complications minor and uncommon.

Unable to succeed consistently with established techniques, the senior author developed a new approach consisting of a continuous excision of excess skin from the arm through the axilla and onto the chest in the form of the letter "L" [5]. Since 2001, this technique has met with consistent success in more than 50 patients, with only minor occasional complication. The "L" represents the shape of the excision, with the long limb along the medial axis of the upper arm and the short limb meeting at right angles across the axilla along the midlateral chest. The sweeping scar across the axilla resembles the letter "L" on its side. The L brachioplasty is designed for the perfuse weight loss deformity, but it can be adapted to the aging arm.

This review of our experience describes the deformity, the marking, the execution, and the integration of the L brachioplasty into upper body lift and breast reshaping surgery. Illustrative results are presented. The discussion elaborates on the rationale and contrasts it with current recognized techniques.

[a] University of Pittsburgh Medical School, Pittsburgh, PA
[b] Magee-Women's Hospital, Pittsburgh, PA
[c] University of Pittsburgh Medical Center, Pittsburgh, PA
* Corresponding author. 3109 Forbes Avenue, Suite 500, Pittsburgh, PA.
E-mail address: drhurwitz@hurwitzcenter.com (D.J. Hurwitz).

doi:10.1016/j.cps.2007.08.005

Deformity

Because the deformity of the upper arm across the axilla onto the chest varies according to the magnitude of original and residual adipose and elastic tissue and transverse skin adherences, there is considerable variability and unique presentations. Nevertheless, there are five consistent distortions in the brachioplasty candidate (Figs. 1 and 2). Results are seen in Figs. 3 and 4.

While our attention is directed to the skin and superficial fat issues, we should recognize that there are underlying musculoskeletal aberrations of unknown impact. The barrel chest rib cage and hypertrophied humerus remain after weight loss. There are oversized superficial flat muscles, such as the latissimus dorsi and pectoralis major. After wide skin excisions and tight closure of an upper body lift, the impact on shortening these muscles is unknown. This complex deformity can be divided into five components.

The first and most outstanding component is the sagging of the upper arm along the posterior margin from the axilla to the elbow. The descent is greatest about the midpoint. The slack posterior arm ranges from loose and wrinkled skin to a thick, unyielding, dangling mass. The anterior arm does not demonstrate these problems because of the lesser effect of gravity and different anatomic adherences. The bicipital groove divides the anterior and posterior compartments of the arm. Medially, the groove is a well-defined, skin-to-fascia adherence leading to an intermuscular septation between the biceps and biceps brachii muscles. Laterally, a less-defined fascia-to-skin adherence continues between the biceps and triceps muscles. The skin anterior to these grooves is diffusely adherent to underlying muscular fascia, whereas skin posterior has a more tenuous attachment. Surgical closure precisely along the medial intermuscular septum can lead to depression of the linear scar line, drawing attention to itself. Likewise, a linear scar along the posterior line may impart a tight sensation, particularly during animation. A posterior scar may flatten the natural rounding around the posterior arm. We believe that the optimal scar starts near the medial epicondyle and ascends the inner arm obliquely to cross the medial bicipital groove in the proximal third on its way to the upper portion of the axilla.

The second abnormality is inferior dislocation of the posterior axillary fold (PAF). The PAF is the posterior skin ridge of the axilla that joins the posterior margin of arm to the chest. The PAF continues along the posterior axillary line of the chest by the lateral border of the latissimus dorsi muscle. The descendent PAF broadens the attachment of the arm to the chest, imparting a disconcerting winglike appearance to the upper arm. The loosely suspended PAF contrasts starkly to the neighboring tightly adherent skin of the deep axillary dome and the elongated and flattened anterior axillary fold.

The third component is the enlarged and cavernous axilla, which we call hyperaxilla. There is enlargement of the normal hair-bearing axillary skin, which is broadly adherent to the underlying retaining clavipectoral fascia canopy. This fascia forms the lateral border of the axilla, which contains major neurovasculature, fat, and lymph nodes. The clavipectoral fascia is retracted after weight loss. Normally, the axillary dome appears deepest with the arm abducted to 90°. Full (180°) abduction of the arm effaces the armpit, but an unnatural depression, and, at times, wavy skin, persists in the patient

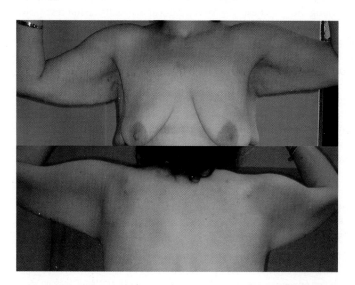

Fig. 1. Unmarked preoperative frontal and posterior views of the upper arms and chest showing moderately severe deformity in a 35-year-old woman. Before her body contouring, she was 5'7" and weighed 157 lbs (BMI 26 kg/m²), having lost 150 lbs 2 years after her Roux-en-Y bypass surgery. She demonstrates sagging upper arm skin, descent of the posterior axillary fold, oversized axilla, elongated and flattened anterior axillary folds, and upper lateral chest roll.

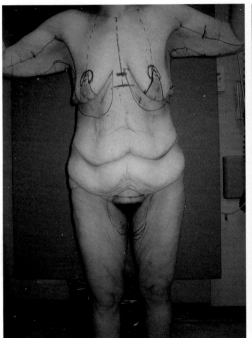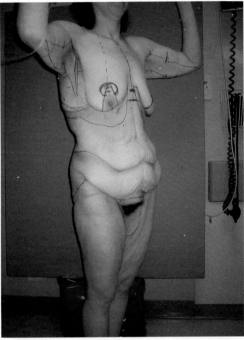

Fig. 2. Full body anterior and right anterior oblique views of the patient in **Fig. 1** with immediate preoperative surgical markings for a total body lift, including the L brachioplasty.

who has had massive weight loss. Arm pit seductiveness relies, in part, on these eye-catching topographic shifts with movement. The weight loss condition obliterates this subtlety. The excessively deep and ever-persistent dome is unsatisfactory to the beholder.

The fourth deformity is the flattened and elongated anterior axillary fold (AAF). The AAF is a ridge

formed along the lateral border of the pectoralis major muscle. As such, it begins at the pectoralis humeral insertion and ends at the superior-lateral breast. The defatted skin does not esthetically reflect the underlying relaxed superficial pectoral muscle, and only slightly more so when the muscle is contracted. The descended breast accentuates the deformity by elongating the unattractive flatness between

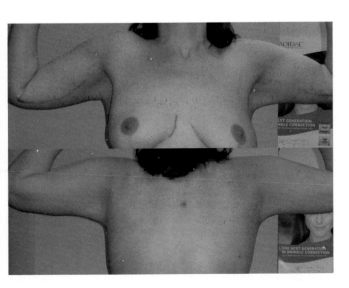

Fig. 3. and 4. Frontal and posterior views of the upper arms and chest (see **Fig. 3**) and right anterior oblique and raised arm full body frontal (see **Fig. 4**) views of the patient shown in **Figs. 1 and 2** 1 year after total body lift and L brachioplasty. The upper arm sagging is corrected symmetrically, leaving a normal drape to the posterior contour. The armpit is smaller and shallower. The posterior axillary fold is raised to the proper position. With the help of the spiral flap reshaping of the breast, the lateral convexity of her breast transitions to a softly reverse curving and shortened anterior axillary fold. The short limb scar of the L is hidden behind the anterior axillary fold, leading to a zigzag unrestrictive crossing of the axilla and curving toward the posterior border of the arm.

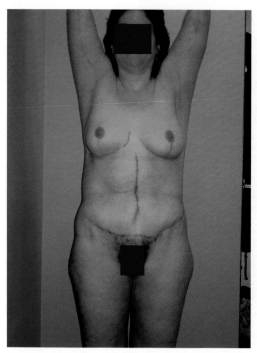

Fig. 4. Postoperative view of patient in Figs. 1–3 with arms fully extended reveal no constricting scars across the axillas.

the clavicle and lateral breast. The desirable "S"-shaped curve descending from the upper anterior arm across the chest and along the lateral breast is stretched to an unappealing "J" in the standing woman. The pleasing contour transitions of the lateralized breast to the axilla in the reclining woman with an outstretched arm are lost. The usual mastopexy and implant augmentation do not reestablish these sensual poses.

The fifth component is the lateral chest skin laxity leading into midtorso transverse rolls. The short limb of the L brachioplasty must be reconciled with the breast reshaping and the effacement of these lateral midtorso rolls. We find it advantageous to perform this complex interaction in a single stage. In other words, crafting the short limb of the L brachioplasty is the last step when combining the brachioplasty with an upper body lift and spiral flap reshaping of the breast. The exception is when a modified Pitanguy lateral thoracoplasty is performed.

Patient selection and goals

The ideal deformity is ptotic and loosely hanging skin that more than doubles the width of the upper arm. Arms oversized with fat need liposuction concurrently or as a preliminary stage if excessive. Extensive liposuction may be too damaging to

remaining skin connective tissue for safe, tight closure.

Patient selection is based on the usual decision making in cosmetic surgery, with special caution on the visibility and unpredictability of the scars. The trade-off of deformity versus surgery with scars along the arm and through the axilla on to the chest must be understood, along with the risk for delayed healing, under- and overresection, wound dehiscence, infection and seromas, and lymphoceles. The deformity in the patient who has sustained massive weight loss usually is so severe as to warrant surgery. We advise that we are seeking an 80% to 90% correction, because 100% skin reduction hazards limb-threatening constriction secondary to the postoperative swelling. Less than desired reduction or recurrent sagging is treated as an office procedure under local anesthesia. Scar hypertrophy or contracture beyond 2 years and aggressive medical treatment usually are treated with surgical revision, which may include a Z-plasty.

The patient needs to appreciate the artistic goals. The arm will be considerably smaller with minimal sagging of the skin. The greatest width will be in the center, with gradual narrow tapering toward the elbow and axilla. The armpit will no longer be too deep and oversized. The skin rolls lateral to the breasts will be effaced. The initially thickened medial arm scar gradually will lighten and thin over several years, with the distal part near the elbow being the last to mature.

This article does not discuss a variety of special situations, such as the arm with oversized adiposity, probably best treated with first-stage liposuction; minimal skin ptosis treated exclusively with liposuction; transverse ringlike constrictions that may need Z-plasty releases; or extension down the medial forearm for distal skin ptosis.

Operative technique

The plan is to excise excess skin and fat of the upper arm through the axilla on to the midlateral chest in the form of an inverted "L," with the closed angle at the dome of the axilla (Figs. 5–8). With the arm abducted, the two elliptical limbs lie perpendicular. When the arm is raised, the ellipses form a straight line, with a gentle zigzag across the axilla. The long ellipse is situated along the medial aspect of the arm. The short ellipse is along the inner half of the axilla and lateral chest.

The goal of the markings is to expeditiously excise nearly all of the excess skin and fat to obtain symmetric effective closures. There should be little adjustment made, except in the obese arm, where excision judgments are particularly hard to make. The markings are made in an obsessively consistent

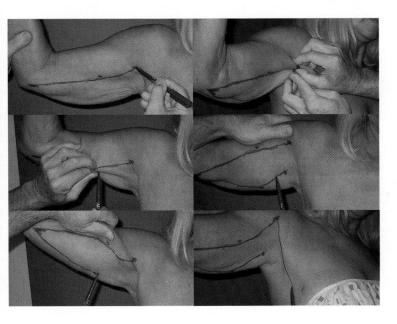

Fig. 5. Preoperative markings for an L brachioplasty in a 59-year-old woman (no weight loss) are made with the arm extended 90° and the forearm flexed 90°. (*Upper left*) A line joins three points from the medial epicondyle, midarm bicipital groove, and deltopectoral groove. (*Middle left*) At the widest sagging of the midarm, the skin is gathered and pinched closed and an inferior mark is made. (*Lower left*) The inferior line is drawn from the epicondyle to the inferior resection mark. (*Upper right*) The elevation of the posterior axillary fold is estimated and marked by gathering lower skin to the deltopectoral mark and straightening the inferior line. (*Middle right*) The inferior incision line continues to that mark. (*Lower right*) A vertical line roughly bisects the axilla to the midlateral chest.

manner. Done in this way, confidence is gained in their accuracy. With the patient sitting, one arm and forearm are abducted 90° with the palm forward as if taking an oath. Do not extend the arm at the elbow because that distorts upper arm skin position. Consistent arm position during marking is essential for accuracy.

Start by marking the midpoint of the arm slightly posterior to the medial bicipital groove. Then, a line is drawn from the medial elbow through the first mark to the deltopectoral groove across the dome of the axilla. There should be a gentle rise to the line; if not, the original midpoint drops a centimeter or so posteriorly. By gathering and pinching excess skin and fat posterior to the initial mark, the width of the midarm excision is determined, and a dot is made near the posterior border of the arm. A straight line is drawn from that point to meet the medial elbow termination of the first line. Then, a critical point is picked and marked along the inferior border of the medial arm that can be pinched approximated across the axilla to the deltopectoral groove. Approximation of this point should raise the PAF adequately and equalize the lengths of the superior and inferior lines. This maneuver may take several attempts to ensure the proper location of this point. The line then angles acutely to descend inferiorly through the axilla, lying away from the PAF. A parallel line descends from the deltopectoral groove through the axilla. The area between these last two lines removes the excess skin of the axilla and lateral chest.

Next, the arm is raised fully to confirm the equal lengths of the inferior and superior incision lines of the upper arm before they zigzag across the axilla and down the lateral chest. In essence, the superior incision of the arm ellipse rises from the medial elbow across the bicipital groove to the deltopectoral groove. The inferior incision of the arm ellipse runs from the medial elbow along the posterior margin of the arm to rise toward the midaxilla. The area between these incisions incorporates the excess skin of the upper arm as determined by tissue-gathering estimates. When there is fatty excess, one has to

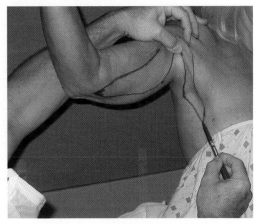

Fig. 6. While the posterior axillary fold triangular flap is pulled toward the deltopectoral groove, the axillary and chest excision lines are completed.

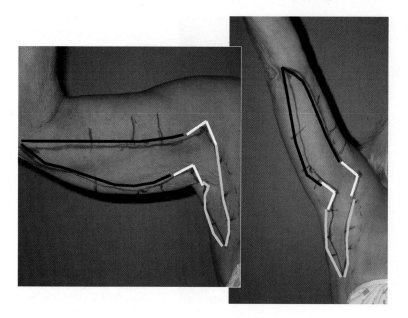

Fig. 7. The final posterior chest lines are drawn, completing the L brachioplasty. As demonstrated by the equal-length white, blue, and yellow lines, excision of the inverted V of axillary skin and advancement of the posterior fold triangular flap causes even incision line approximation with a zigzag across the axilla.

consider the volume reduction that will be due to liposuction. The second ellipse drops vertically from the deltopectoral groove to remove approximately the medial half of the axilla and continues vertically to include excess lateral chest wall skin. The chest portion of this ellipse is coordinated with the transverse removal of a back roll performed during an upper body lift.

An inferiorly based triangular flap of the proximal posterior upper arm has been formed as the inferior arm incision meets the lateral incision of the vertically oriented axillary ellipse. The ability

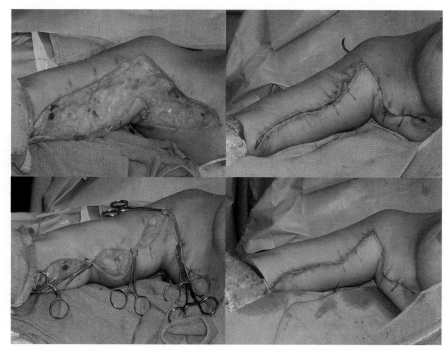

Fig. 8. Intraoperative views showing the right arm of the patient seen in Figs. 5–7 on an arm board on the operating room table with the skin and superficial fat excised in the form of an inverted L, followed by deep running absorbable skin closure.

to advance this triangular flap to the deltopectoral groove is confirmed by pinch approximation. This maneuver elevates the ptotic PAF, with tapering of the arm skin toward the axilla. The markings are reevaluated with the arm and forearm extended fully above the head. The arm and chest ellipses should have lengths that are equal to their limbs. Cross-hatching alignment lines are drawn while the arm is outstretched upwardly.

The operation

With the patient supine, the arms are abducted 80° on operating room table arm boards (see Fig. 8). Arm intravenous infusion is avoided to prevent swelling that is due to fluid extravasation. The arms are prepped with antiseptic from midforearm to midlateral chest. The unprepped forearm, with a forearm blood pressure cuff, is wrapped in sterile drapes. The width of arm skin resection is checked one more time. If there is any doubt about safe closure, a slightly narrower ellipse is drawn. Several hundred milliliters of saline with 1 mg of epinephrine and 20 mL of 1% xylocaine per liter are infused until the tissues are firm. After waiting about 10 minutes for vasoconstriction, lipoplasty is performed. Ultrasonic-assisted lipoplasty is preferred because of maximal vascular and connective tissue preservation. The fat under the ellipse in the arm is removed as completely as possible, leaving a depressed area for resection of skin only. Limited suction lipoplasty may be performed in areas not planned for resection.

With the medial skin rolled superiorly, the inferior incision is made with a scalpel through skin to the superficial fascia. With the tension applied, the properly incised wound literally splits open like an overboiled hot dog. Then, the posterior arm skin is undermined about 1 cm. Hemostasis is obtained by grasping vessels and applying electrocautery. After one final check for the suitability of the excision, the arching superior incision is made from the elbow to the deltopectoral groove. The anterior skin edge also is undermined minimally, being sure to leave subcutaneous fascia. Usually, there is little bleeding.

Next, the outline of the shorter axillary–chest ellipse is incised. The incisions are no deeper than the dermis in the axilla, whereas in the chest the incisions extend through fat to serratus fascia. If a spiral flap breast shaping is to be performed, the posterior limb of the ellipse is not incised until the mastopexy/augmentation is completed. Less width of skin may need to be taken because the added fill to the breast will take up lateral chest skin excess.

The resection starts with grasping the distal end of the arm skin ellipse with a sharp pointed clamp or rake. This instrument firmly distracts the ellipse up and toward the chest as a full-thickness, skin graftlike resection is cut with a scalpel. The subdermal connective tissue with vasculature and nerves is detached sharply from the skin being removed. Bleeding is minimal. The level of excision is subdermal through the axilla and then completed deeply over muscular fascia of the lateral chest. The clavipectoral fascia of the axilla is seen, but not entered. Major veins and sensory nerves are not seen; instead, there is a latticework of connective tissue nearly empty of adipose. The skin is discarded only when closure is complete.

Using the previously drawn hatchmarks, the incisions are aligned with towel hooks. A larger interrupted absorbable suture anchors the subcutaneous fascia of the triangular flap across the axilla to the deltoid fascia. A continuous running 2-0 gauge long-lasting, but absorbable, suture approximates the subcutaneous fascia. We prefer using a running 2-0 braided absorbable, such as Vicryl (Ethicon, Somerville, New Jersey) or Polysorb (U. S. Surgical, Norwalk, Connecticut). We also have successfully run the double-ended barbed suture by Quill (Angiotech, Vancouver, British Columbia), thereby having a secure closure with no knots. We prefer absorbable braided suture because it can be cinched and tightened as it is placed. If the approximation of the wound edges opens, an assistant pulls on the thread or the edges are held together with a towel clip. As the suturing approaches a towel clip, a second clip leap frogs ahead before that clamp is released. A second smaller-caliber continuous monofilament intradermal closure follows. Dermal glue completes the operation. No drains are used. The operative time for both arms is approximately 90 minutes, but frequently the time was halved by team surgery.

The arms are wrapped in gauze and an ace wrap. The arms are elevated on several pillows and raised even higher, and the elastic wraps may be removed upon excessive swelling of the hands. If the V-shaped flap in the axilla has good color at 3 days, the ace wraps are exchanged for elastic, long-sleeved garments.

With resolution of the edema and equilibration of the skin tensions, the scar settles between the bicipital groove and posterior edge of the arm. It rises gently to the axillary dome and then drops vertically through the midaxilla to the lateral chest, forming an inverted "L." With arms at the side, the scars should not be visible. With the arms raised, the scar unobtrusively crosses the axilla without contracture. There is no drifting of the scar from the axilla to the arm, probably because of the broad adherence of the advanced triangular flap to the axilla.

The arm contour tapers normally from the center outward, leading into a smooth-skinned axilla of proper depth and dimensions. The inferior contour of the arm drops slightly at the midhumerus and then rises distinctly to a superiorly positioned PAF. The suspended PAF skin adheres fully to the reduced-in-size axillary hollow. The skin along the midlateral chest is smooth and adherent, with a defined and roundly sensuous border with the lateral breast. When a spiral flap breast reshaping is done, the flattened and elongated AAF is filled and curvaceous (see Figs. 3, 4, and 9).

Most of our more than 50 patients are pleased. All arms were closed primarily without dehiscence. Tip necrosis of the V-advancement flap occurred in about 20% of the cases. This problem decreased by withholding the early use of elastic sleeves. Debridement in the axilla and secondary closure was needed in 3 patients. Another patient required skin grafting of delayed healing axillary and hip wounds. Further limited skin reduction was performed after a year in 2 patients. One obese patient suffered chronic mild total arm swelling that was temporarily responsive to pressure therapy. Recurrent lymphoceles of 3 to 5 cm in the mid to distal medial arm occurred in about 20% of the patients. All lymphoceles responded to repeated aspiration and localized pressure. A few patients live with walnut-sized lumps.

The senior author believed that all patients were greatly improved, but that the arms of some of the severe cases were still slightly too large, although the wound closures were tight. Most patients wear sleeveless tops in the summer because their scars are not visible unless the arms are outstretched. All patients were pleased by their shallower, smaller, and smoother axillas.

Complete maturation of the scars often took longer than 2 years, so patients should be encouraged to wait extended periods for scar fade. No patient expressed regret over the trade-off for one's inner arm scar. The axillary scars were faint and a nonissue in all but a few patients. There was persistent banding from the axilla to the chest in several patients, leading to two Z-plasties.

Discussion

Following massive weight loss, women develop bizarre arm deformity that extends through the axilla and on to the chest. We found prevalent full-length brachioplasties inadequate to fully treat this deformity [1–4]. Furthermore, the straight scars along the bicipital groove or along the posterior border were too conspicuous. Ending the linear scar into Ts or Zs upon entry into the axilla did not improve esthetics.

The L brachioplasty is designed for the deformities of the upper arm, axilla, and lateral chest of the patient who has sustained massive weight loss. It also seems to be applicable to the aged arm. Because both types of patients have hanging skin and poor elasticity, pulling skin from a distance is ineffective. Short-scar techniques are inadequate [6–8]. In most cases, excess skin needs to be removed along the entire length of the arm. The challenge is how to do this simply, symmetrically, and reliably, leaving esthetic contours and scars. Furthermore, the hyperaxilla, descended PAF, and lateral chest roll need attention.

The width of the excisions through the arm and chest wall is based on preoperative assessment of excess skin through anatomic point locations followed by pinch-and-gathering maneuvers. With consistent and careful marking technique, adequacy of resection, proper scar location, and symmetry are expected. As advocated by other

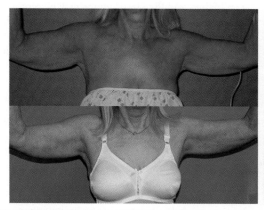
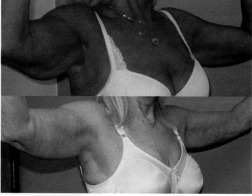

Fig. 9. (*Upper*) Frontal and oblique views of the patient in Figs. 5 through 8 before and 2 years after L brachioplasty. (*Lower*) The symmetric improvement of the arm skin sag, smoothing and reduction of the axilla, and reduction of a lateral chest roll. The arm scar rises slowly from the posterior elbow to the axillary dome and then bisects the anterior and posterior axillary folds. There is no scar depression or contracture.

investigators [9], preformed skin excision patterns play no role.

The geometry of the L-shaped excision spanning the upper arm, axilla, and lateral chest is designed uniquely to deal with incision lines of predictably uneven length and the advancement of the PAF triangular flap into the axilla (see Fig. 3). The superior incision line of the arm (along the bicipital groove) is shorter than is the inferior incision line along the sagging posterior border, because the excess skin hangs like a hammock between the axilla and elbow. The arm skin excision is more like a hemi-ellipse than a true ellipse. Likewise, there is more sagging skin along the posterior axillary line than the anterior line, creating another hemi-ellipse. Joining these arm and lateral chest skin excisions is an inverted V-shape of skin to be removed from the axilla. The inverted-V excision allows cephalic advancement of a triangular flap of PAF to the deltopectoral junction. By advancing this flap, the superior and inferior arm incisions and the anterior and lateral chest incision lengths are equalized. The equal length of these lines is clearer with the arm in a hyperextended position. Closure is along the preoperative hatch marks, requiring no intraoperative length, dog ear, or Z-plasty adjustments.

Many operative techniques include Z-plasty or fish tail adjustments through the axilla to retard scar contracture [1,10–13]. That is a conceptual error, because the axillary deformity is addressed secondarily. Therefore, esthetic improvement of the armpit is unlikely. The Z-plasty triangular flaps may interpose different quality skin (hair bearing, nonhair bearing, thin, and thick), which leaves an unnatural—and sometimes cobblestone-like—appearance. The ill fit relates to the static Z-shaped scar in a dynamically reshaped armpit and the subtle coning at each closed angle of the Z-plasty. The rare scar hypertrophy after a Z-plasty leaves an unmistakable surgical geometric branding. In the unusual instance of scar contracture across the axilla following an L brachioplasty, it can be treated secondarily with an ideally positioned Z-plasty immediately inferior to the axilla.

Alternatively, there are T-plasty excisions with limited elevation of the descended PAF [3,14]. This technique leaves two right-angle arm flaps leading into the axilla. Tip necrosis with widened scars and contracture does occur. The T-junction may drift unesthetically into the arm.

Leaving a lazy L-shaped scar obscures the scar appearance and retards contracture. The medial arm scar rises gently from the distal posterior arm to the apex of the axilla, thwarting the tendency of contracture when it lies totally within the bicipital groove. The operation is simple in design and executed rapidly. If obesity makes the resection width difficult to assess, be conservative in the resection and resect more skin or suction more fat after approximating the skin edges with towel clips late in the operation. Alternatively, the procedure can be performed with segmental cutting and checking; however, we believe that the decision about the right amount to remove is best made preoperatively, before fluid infusions and intraoperative swelling. If intraoperative swelling is too great, the arm may be wrapped and closed some days later.

After designing the L brachioplasty, the senior author learned of Pitanguy's extended brachioplasty through the axilla onto the chest and under the breast [15]. Unlike Pitanguy's technique, the L brachioplasty's anterior incision line is made just behind the AAF. This position allows greatest effect to raise the descended PAF. Competing wound edge tension pulls the ultimate scar to the midlateral chest. Pitanguy made little note of improvement of the axilla. In fact, plastic surgeons have ignored the esthetics of the axilla and upper lateral chest.

The cutaneous axilla (armpit) is a dome-shaped structure formed by the tight adherence of thin, mostly hair-bearing axillary skin to the suspending clavipectoral fascia. The axilla is bordered by the inner arm, lateral chest, and axillary folds. The AAF (AAF) is created by skin adherence to the lateral edge of the pectoralis major muscle. The gentle concavity of the AAF turns abruptly convex around the lateral border of the breast. The posterior border is the PAF, created by skin adherence along the lateral edge of the latissimus dorsi muscle. Atrophy or resection of these muscles disrupts these folds. Unseen with the arms at the side, the armpit crevasse is seductively deepest when the arm is extend 90° degrees and undulating contours with the arm raised fully. Along with the spiral flap reshaping of the breast, the L brachioplasty restores these complex esthetic curves [16,17].

Troublesome postoperative lymphedema and lymphoceles complicate brachioplasty [18]. Pascal's [19] logic of extensive, lymphatic-sparing, preexcision liposuction and his excellent results have encouraged us to do the same in recent cases. We prefer preexcision ultrasonic-assisted lipoplasty to traditional lipoplasty. Out of a dozen or so treated patients, one small nonaspirated lymphocele has occurred in a distal upper arm. The deep subcutaneous nerves also should be avoided, particularly the medial brachiocutaneous along the distal arm [18]. The L brachioplasty also can be performed without liposuction.

The scalpel excision of skin only after liposuction preserves the underlying vasculature. The closure is a running absorbable suture into the poorly developed subcutaneous fascia. Since the triangular flap is secured to deltoid fascia, there is no need to anchor it to axillary fascia, which may injure major nerves [3,13]. The advanced PAF skin smoothly conforms to the hemi-dome of the axilla.

An appreciation of the esthetic arm contour unravels the weight loss arm deformity. Arm reduction that amputates the inferior excess from the medial and lateral side destroys the natural midarm drape and accentuates the still ptotic PAF. The midposterior arm becomes flat and tight just where it should be curved and soft. Posterior scars tend to contract noticeably [2].

The L brachioplasty restores these anatomic subtleties in patients who have sustained weight loss and in aging patients with the least obtrusive scar. The success is due to the large resection of skin and the direct triangular flap advancement of the axillary fold. There are no geometric scars or dog ears from rotation flaps.

Summary

The L-shaped brachioplasty is an innovative, effective, reliable, esthetic, and safe technique following massive weight loss. The upper arm skin excess is reduced, leaving a tapered junction to a raised PAF. Arm mobility is unrestricted with an inconspicuous scar across the axilla. Integrating the brachioplasty into the upper body lift improves the contours of the axilla, breast, and upper lateral chest, contributing to improved harmonious body contour. The L brachioplasty also has succeeded for selected aging cases.

References

[1] Regnault P. Brachioplasty, axilloplasty, and pre-axilloplasty. Aesthetic Plast Surg 1983;7:31–6.

[2] Vogt PA, Baroudi R. Brachioplasty and brachial suction-assisted lipectomy. In: Cohen M, editor. Mastery of plastic and reconstructive surgery. Boston: Little Brown and Co; 1994. p. 2219–36.

[3] Lockwood T. Brachioplasty with superficial fascial system suspension. Plast Reconstr Surg 1995;96:912–20.

[4] Baroudi R. Dermolipectomy of the upper arm. Clin Plast Surg 1975;2:485–91.

[5] Hurwitz DJ, Holland SW. The L brachioplasty: an innovative approach to correct excess tissue of the upper arm, axilla and lateral chest. Plast Reconstr Surg 2006;117(2):403–11.

[6] Temourian B. Rejuvenation of the upper arm. Plast Reconstr Surg 1998;102:545–52.

[7] Richards ME. Minimal-incision brachioplasty: a first-choice option in arm reduction surgery. Aesth Surg J 2001;21:301–10.

[8] Abramson DL. Minibrachioplasty: minimizing scars while maximizing results. Plast Reconstr Surg 2004;114:1631–4.

[9] de Souza Pinto EB, Erazo PJ, Matsuda CA, et al. Rejuvenation technique with the use of molds. Plast Reconstr Surg 2000;105:1854–60.

[10] Guerrerosantos J. Brachioplasty. Aesthetic Plast Surg 1979;3:1–9.

[11] Regnault P. Brachioplasty, axilloplasty, and pre-axilloplasty. Presented at VII International Congress of the Confederation of Plastic and Reconstructive Surgery. Rio de Janeiro, May 20–25, 1979.

[12] Chandawarker RY, Lewis JM. "Fish-incision" brachioplasty. J Plast Reconstr Aesthet Surg 2006; 59(5):521–5.

[13] Strauch B. A technique of brachioplasty. Plast Reconstr Surg 2004;113:1044–52.

[14] Juri J, Juri C, Elias J. Arm dermolipectomy with a quadrangular flap and "T" closure. Plast Reconstr Surg 1979;64(4):521–5.

[15] Pitanguy I. Correction of lipodystrophy of the lateral thoracic aspect and inner side of the arm and elbow. Clin Plast Surg 1975;2: 477–83.

[16] Hurwitz DJ. Single stage total body lift after massive weight loss. Ann Plast Surg 2004;52(5): 435–41.

[17] Hurwitz DJ, Agha-Mohammadi S. Post bariatric surgery breast reshaping: the spiral flap. Ann Plast Surg 2006;56(5):481–6.

[18] Knoetgen J. Long-term outcomes and complications associated with brachioplasty: a retrospective review and cadaveric study. Plast Reconstr Surg 2006;117(7):2219–23.

[19] Pascal JF. Brachioplasty. Aesthetic Plast Surg 2005;29:423–9.

ELSEVIER
SAUNDERS

CLINICS IN
PLASTIC
SURGERY

Clin Plastic Surg 35 (2008) 141–147

Brachioplasty in the Massive Weight Loss Patient

Al Aly, MD, FACS[a],*, Shehab Soliman, MD[b], Albert Cram, MD, FACS[a]

- Presentation and patient selection
- Treatment
  Markings
  Surgical technique
  Segmental resection-closure surgical
    technique
- Postoperative care
- Results
  Complications
- Summary
- References

The lower truncal subunit is the area most often first treated in the patient who has achieved massive weight loss. Another area that is extremely bothersome for many of these patients is the upper arm. Deformities of the upper arm vary in their presentation from minor deformities to rather extensive excess skin of the upper arms. Obviously the treatment should be adjusted to the extent of the presenting deformity. Certainly, if the quality of skin is good and the extent of excess is rather minimal, traditional techniques can be used. The technique discussed in this article should be reserved for extensive excess skin in the upper arm.

Presentation and patient selection

Patients who have sustained massive weight loss present to the plastic surgeon in a variety of ways. In some patients the arms will have not been affected to any great degree by the weight gain/loss process. Others will present with arms that are significantly over-inflated despite stabilization of weight loss. For those patients the authors recommend a staged initial liposuction procedure to deflate the arms to an appropriate level before performing an excisional procedure, usually 6 months later. The ideal patient on whom to perform an excisional procedure

presents with deflated arms. Another group of patients present with intermediate amounts of retained fat, and patient and surgeon together must decide whether to pursue a direct course to excisional resection or to undertake a staged approach, as described for over-inflated arms.

As with any deformity to be treated by plastic surgery, an understanding of the nature of upper arm deformity in the patient who has sustained massive weight loss is imperative to design a surgical approach for treatment. Careful examination and observation of these deformities has revealed that the excess is located in the posterior axillary fold and its extension down the arm, Fig. 1.

Thus the excess of the upper arm in patients who have sustained massive weight loss crosses from the arm to the axilla at the posterior axillary fold and onto the lateral chest wall.

Treatment

The authors' surgical approach for the treatment of upper arm deformities is based on a few important principles:

- **Because the upper arm excess crosses the axilla, the surgical resection must cross the axilla.**

[a] Iowa City Plastic Surgery, 501 12th Avenue, Suite 102, Coralville, Iowa 52241, USA
[b] Department of Surgery, Cairo University, Kasr El-Aini Hospitals, Cairo, Egypt
* Corresponding author.
E-mail address: mdplastic@aol.com (A. Aly).

doi:10.1016/j.cps.2007.09.004

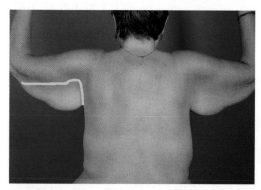

Fig. 1. Excess of the upper arm crosses the axilla onto the lateral chest wall in most massive weight loss patients.

- Brachioplasty is a resection of tissue around a cylinder with a noncompressible musculoskeletal inner core.
- Efficiency in surgical time is critical when performing brachioplasty resections if aggressive but appropriate resections are desired.

Markings

The meticulous and precise marking based on the surgical plan is a cornerstone to attain a successful outcome of the operation. It is preferred to do the markings 1 day before surgery to allow time to photograph the markings adequately, evaluate them, and, if needed, adjust them before surgery. Because patients present with varying degrees of deformity, it is important to digest the principles underlying the marking process. Equipped with this knowledge, each surgeon can create his or her marking sequence.

The double-ellipse marking technique

The upper arm is marked for brachioplasty using the two-ellipse technique. It comprises an outer ellipse based on anatomic reference points that follow the extent of the upper arm deformity across the axilla and onto the lateral chest wall and/or the elbow, if needed. An inner ellipse is based on the outer one but is adjusted to allow closure around the cylindrical upper arm. It is important to understand that, when using the pinch test to estimate the amount of excess tissue in the arm, the surgeon must account for the distance between his or her examining fingers.

The patient is marked while sitting on a swivel chair while the surgeon stands at the patient's side. The axillary crease level is identified first by adducting and abducting the patient's arm to determine the break point. With the arm abducted to 90° and starting from the axillary crease, the pinch technique is used to make anterior and posterior marks

along the upper arm. The same process is performed on the lateral chest wall along the posterior axillary fold. The extent to which the markings extend onto the arm or the lateral chest wall is dictated by the amount of excess. Sometimes it is necessary to cross the elbow, but the authors prefer not to cross by more than 5 to 8 cm. Joining these points creates the outer ellipse. Attempting to excise this ellipse probably will result in an inability to close the defect created because of failure to account for the distance between the pinching fingers. To make an adjustment for this distance, a second ellipse is marked inside the first that allows enough skin to be left behind to span the distance between the pinching fingers [1]. For example, if the distance between the pinching fingers is 2 cm, then the marks for the new ellipse are moved in 1 cm on each side (Fig. 2).

This adjustment is made all along the arm component of the first ellipse but not on the chest wall component, because once the excision reaches the lateral chest wall, the tissues can be undermined, if need be (undermining is dangerous and nonproductive on the arm). Joining the adjustment points creates the inner ellipse. Crosshatch marks are made to help alignment at closure, and a central line is drawn to approximate the position of the final scar (Fig. 3) [1].

Surgical technique

If brachioplasty is going to be performed alone, it can be performed with the patient in the supine position with both arms prepped and draped at the same time. If the procedure is part of an upper body lift, the patient is turned to one of the lateral decubitus positions and padded appropriately. In either case, the markings are reinforced by methylene blue hatch-mark tattoos. The authors prefer to inject the proposed wound edges of the inner ellipse with a local anesthetic solution containing epinephrine to reduce incisional bleeding. The patient then is prepped and draped. At this point another check is performed to confirm the feasibility of using the proposed inner ellipse marks as the extents of excision. The inner ellipse marks are tailor-tacked with staples. If any areas along the entire resection line seem to be too tight, the marks are adjusted, Fig. 4.

Segmental resection-closure surgical technique

Because of the cylindrical nature of the arm, with its noncompressible inner musculoskeletal core, small amounts of edema generated by surgical manipulation between the skin and the inner core can prevent closure of a nicely estimated resection. Thus

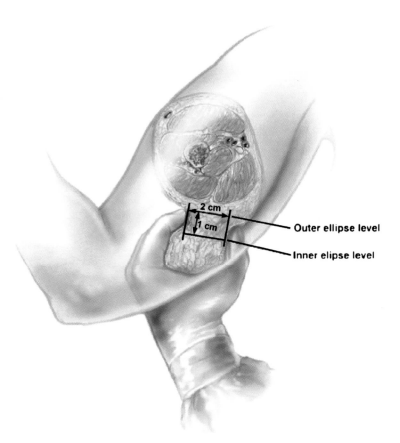

2 cm

1 cm

Outer ellipse level

Inner elipse level

Fig. 2. An adjustment is made at each point along the entire upper arm. Thus the inner ellipse is an adjustment to the first ellipse based on the thickness of the pinch. (*From* Aly A, Cram AE, Pace D. Brachioplasty in the patient with massive weight loss. Aesthetic Surg J 2006;26: 76–84; with permission. Copyright © 2006 by The American Society for Aesthetic Plastic Surgery, Inc.)

the authors use a "segmental resection-closure" surgical technique that is designed to eliminate the possibility of being unable to close the arm because of intraoperative edema. The procedure starts distally and proceeds proximally. Retraction clamps are placed along the central line of the inner ellipse. Traction on these clamps facilitates the dissection planes during the resection. Incisions are made on either side of the ellipse up to the first crosshatch mark. The skin with its underlying subcutaneous fat then is dissected as a proximally based flap. The dissection plane is at or just above the level of the underlying muscle fascia. Once the first crosshatch mark is reached, the area of resection is closed temporarily with skin staples. With the staples in place, no significant edema will develop in that segment. The resection then continues to the next segment, and the same pattern of resection is followed (Fig. 5) [1].

If the closure at any segment is considered too tight, the proximally-based skin/fat flap can be introduced partially back into the wound, and the entire resection line can be adjusted (Fig. 6) [2].

When the resection reaches the area straddling the axillary crease, the dissection is performed in a more superficial plane to avoid damage to the

lymphatic structures. Once the entire arm resection is completed and closed with staples, a Z-plasty is performed at axillary crease level to prevent linear contraction of the wound. A closed suction drain is inserted through a separate stab wound at the lateral chest wall and is threaded through the wound as distally as possible. As discussed later, if the brachioplasty is performed as part of an upper body lift in a male, the lateral thoracic wall component is left with temporary staples to allow adjustment during the breast surgery portion of the procedure. The remainder of the arm is closed in two layers. The first layer is a 0-PDS that approximates the deep tissues up to the subdermal level. Although this layer of closure attempts to approximate the superficial fascial system, the fascia in the arm is quite weak and is difficult to delineate or depend on. The skin is closed with either interrupted or running subcuticular 2-0 and 3-0 Monocryl sutures. A layer of skin glue is applied to the closure. No compression garments or wrapping are used acutely.

Postoperative care

If the brachioplasty is performed by itself, the patient can go home the same day. If it is part of an

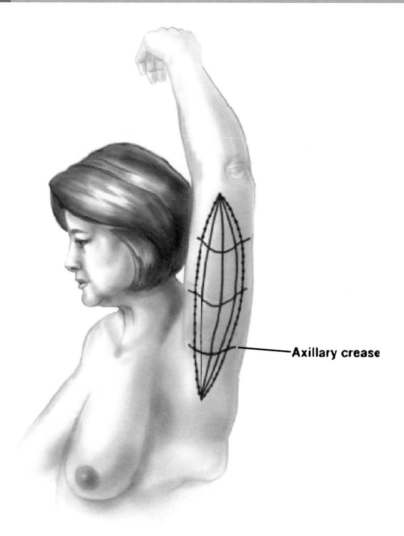

Fig. 3. The double-ellipse markings in place. (*From* Aly A, Cram AE, Pace D. Brachioplasty in the patient with massive weight loss. Aesthetic Surg J 2006;26:76–84; with permission. Copyright © 2006 by The American Society for Aesthetic Plastic Surgery, Inc.)

Axillary crease

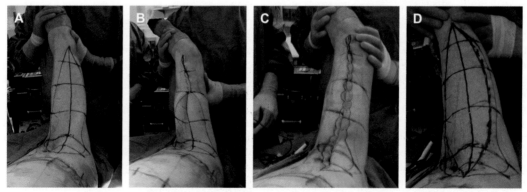

Fig. 4. The sequence of steps performed before making incisions in the operating room. (*A*) The proposed inner ellipse to be excised. (*B, C*) The tailor-tacking at different stages. (*D*) The final adjustments made after the tailor-tacking.

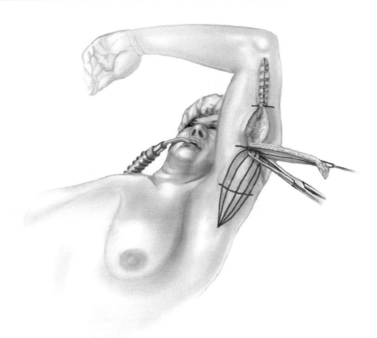

Fig. 5. The segmental resection-closure technique. As each segment is resected, it is closed quickly and temporarily with skin staples to prevent edema from developing in that segment. (*From* Aly A, Cram AE, Pace D. Brachioplasty in the patient with massive weight loss. Aesthetic Surg J 2006;26:76–84; with permission. Copyright © 2006 by The American Society for Aesthetic Plastic Surgery, Inc.)

upper body lift, however, the patient stays in the hospital for 1 night. Arms are kept elevated above the level of the heart in a slightly flexed position for about 3 weeks, except when the patient is eating or going to the bathroom. Drains are removed when discharge is 40 mL or less in a 24-hour period, usually within 4 to 6 days. At 10 to 14 days patients are asked to wear compression garments that start at the hand. The compression is used for 2 to 3 months. The scar will take the usual year to mature and often is thick and raised. It often subsides with time, but overall usually it is the least

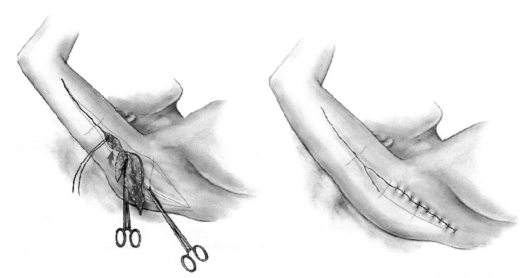

Fig. 6. Adjustments can be made if the resection is deemed to be excessively tight. The proximal area of closure is opened, the proximally based, partly resected flap is partially reintroduced into the wound, and the entire resection line is adjusted to accommodate the appropriate closure. (*From* Aly AS, Cram AE. Brachioplasty. In: Aly AS, editor. Body contouring after massive weight loss. St Louis (MO): Quality Medical Publishing, 2005. p. 303–33; with permission.)

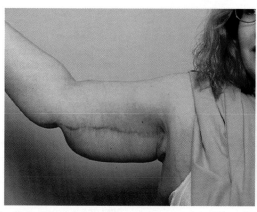
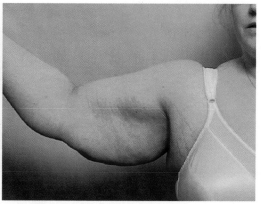

Fig. 7. (*Left*) A patient who underwent a traditional "T" brachioplasty. (*Right*) Note the lack of improvement because the excision does not cross the axilla.

attractive scar that a patient who has had massive weight loss will develop from the various operations he or she undergoes.

Results

The improvement that can be attained by this technique and by most, but not all, techniques that cross the axilla is considerably better than can be attained by more traditional "T" type resections (Figs. 7–9).

One should note that the scar is located at the most inferior point of the abducted arm, not in the bicipital groove. The authors believe that the more posterior position is better because an arm scar is most likely to be revealed during normal, everyday animation, which places the scar in the bicipital groove in an extremely visible position. The position of the scar, however, is a matter of preference that will vary from patient to patient and surgeon to surgeon. Thus there is no absolute correct position for the scar; it is a matter of taste and philosophy.

Complications

Complications that can occur after brachioplasty include small wound separations, dehiscences,

seroma, lymphocele/lymphedema, inability to close the arm, bad scarring, infection, bleeding, nerve compression/compartment syndrome, neuromas, and sensory loss. The problems that occur most often after this technique of brachioplasty are small wound separations at the Z-plasty. The authors have used permanent suture or staples in this area to reinforce the closure for about 2 weeks postoperatively. This precaution has greatly reduced, but has not eliminated, this problem. Significant dehiscences usually result from technical difficulties and usually can be avoided with good technique. Seromas are common after brachioplasty but tend to occur at a later time after surgery, 4 to 6 weeks. It is not clear to the authors why seromas occur, but it might be related to lack of compression; thus the authors try to continue the use of a compression garment use as long as the patient will tolerate it. If a seroma should occur, it usually is aspirated a number of times. If it does not resolve, it is injected with a sclerosing agent a number of times. If this procedure is not successful, exteriorization of the cavity is performed by making a small opening through the scar into the cavity, inserting

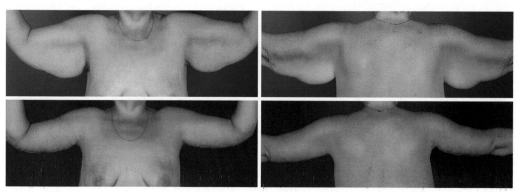

Fig. 8. A patient before (*top*) and after (*bottom*) undergoing the technique presented in this article. Note the significant improvement over Fig. 8.

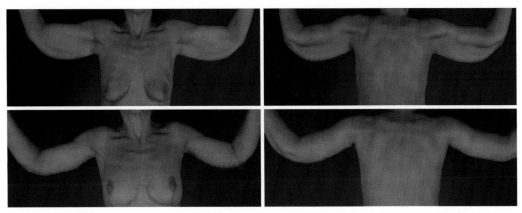

Fig. 9. A second patient before (*top*) and after (*bottom*) the brachioplasty technique described in this article. Note the position of the scar.

a Penrose drain, and leaving the drain in place until the cavity fills itself in and stops draining.

Inability to close the arm after resection is caused either by over-resection of skin or development of intraoperative soft tissue edema . Over-resection of skin can be avoided by careful planning and the intraoperative adjustments discussed in the technique section. If, however, the surgeon deems that there is an over-resection after the entire excision has been completed, some of the resected skin can be harvested as a full-thickness skin graft to be applied to the area of deficiency. Unfortunately this option often results in potential litigation; thus it behooves the surgeon to discuss this possibility with the patient before surgery.

If the surgeon considers that the amount resected is appropriate and the difficulty with closure is caused by intraoperative edema, a few untied sutures can be placed in the area in question, and the arm can be wrapped lightly and raised for a week. The patient then is taken back to the operating room, and the sutures are tied. Even if this outcome is considered likely at the original procedure, the original resected skin should be kept in a frozen state to allow full-thickness skin grafting, should it be required.

The patient may develop nerve compression, usually in the ulnar nerve distribution, either alone or as part of an overall picture of compartment syndrome. The treatment is that which would be in used any such clinical situation.

Neuromas may occur with any brachioplasty technique, although the medial cutaneous antebrachial nerve is located within the resection area of techniques that attempt to place the final scar in the bicipital groove. This nerve, in particular, is less likely to be involved with a neuroma if the technique described in this article is used, because it is not in the field of resection.

Any brachioplasty technique is associated with a certain degree of sensory loss, although the authors are not aware of any studies that have delineated a typical pattern. Empirically, the authors have noted that for 6 months to a year after the surgery, there is a 2- to 3-cm area of sensory loss on either side of the scar. The authors intend to study the pattern of long-term sensory loss prospectively. They also believe that the pattern of loss will be found to depend on the position of scar and the technique used.

Summary

The arm deformity encountered in most patients who have had massive weight loss is severe. The excess crosses the axilla as an extension of the posterior axillary fold. Surgical treatment requires crossing the axilla with the excision. The final scar position is on the posterior aspect of the arm and is more hidden when the person is animating. The authors have found this technique to be powerful and superior to other available techniques.

References

[1] Aly A, Cram AE, Pace D. Brachioplasty in the patient with massive weight loss. Aesthetic Surg J 2006;26:76–84.

[2] Aly AS, Cram AE. Brachioplasty. In: Aly AS, editor. Body contouring after massive weight loss. St Louis (MO): Quality Medical Publishing; 2005. p. 303–33.

ELSEVIER
SAUNDERS

CLINICS IN
PLASTIC
SURGERY

Clin Plastic Surg 35 (2008) 149

Editorial Commentary

The two brachioplasty techniques presented in the last two articles share one very important factor: they both cross the axilla with their respective excisions. This is critical because patients who have undergone massive weight loss present with excess that spans from the upper arm, across the axilla, and onto the lateral chest wall. Any technique that does not account for this will probably not produce the desired results.

The two techniques also have many differences and I would ask the reader to realize that it is human nature to become infatuated with one's own invention (this certainly applies to me). It is thus difficult for authors to be objective about their own work. It is the job of the reader when evaluating techniques to glean the concepts on which the techniques are based, decide if they agree with them, and determine if the results attained are worthy of adoption.

doi:10.1016/j.cps.2007.10.018

ELSEVIER
SAUNDERS

CLINICS IN
PLASTIC
SURGERY

Clin Plastic Surg 35 (2008) 151–163

Current Concepts in Medial Thighplasty

David W. Mathes, MD[a], Jeffrey M. Kenkel, MD[b],*

The medial thigh area remains a troublesome region for body contouring in patients with generalized lipodystrophy and skin flaccidity. Skin laxity is one of the first signs of aging in the thighs and is often a harbinger of significant ptosis in the body. The use of suction-assisted lipectomy to contour the medial thigh is effective in patients with lipodystrophy without skin laxity. However, in most circumstances, this technique fails to remodel and tighten the inner thigh where the skin is often thin and inelastic. Aggressive liposuction may also result in conspicuous contour abnormalities. In many patients, rejuvenation of the medial thigh requires removal of fat deposits as well as excision and re-draping of the medial thigh skin. This is especially true in the massive weight loss (MWL) patient, where skin laxity can be quite severe and extend down to, and even below, the knee.

The medial thigh lift was first described by Lewis [1] more than 30 years ago, but did not gain widespread acceptance because of the postoperative problems of inferior wound migration, widening of the scars, lateral traction deformity of the vulva, and early recurrence of ptosis. The morbidity is due in part to the thin nature of the skin and dermis

and the loss of a well-defined superficial fascial system in the medial thigh. Lockwood [2,3] attempted to address these issues when he described a fascial anchoring technique in the medial thigh lift (Fig. 1). He recommended anchoring the dermal tissue of the distal medial thigh tissue to the Colles' fascia to allow for a more stable and long-term result. These changes in surgical design of the medial thigh lift have improved results and decreased complications but still have the fundamental problem of poor tissue-fixation to rigid tissue.

To provide increased support to the medial thigh incisions, modifications to this technique have been tried. This article describes our approach to the medial thigh lift in both those patients who have undergone weight loss and in the more traditional thigh-lift patient [4–10].

Anatomy

In contradistinction to other areas undergoing surgical rejuvenation, such as the abdomen or the lateral thigh, the medial thigh has a relatively thin dermal component. Under the dermis are two

[a] Division of Plastic Surgery, Department of Surgery, University of Washington School of Medicine, Seattle, WA, USA
[b] Department of Plastic Surgery, The University of Texas Southwestern Medical Center, Dallas, Texas, USA
* Corresponding author.
E-mail address: jeffrey.kenkel@utsouthwestern.edu (J.M. Kenkel).

0094-1298/08/$ – see front matter © 2008 Elsevier Inc. All rights reserved.
plasticsurgery.theclinics.com

doi:10.1016/j.cps.2007.09.003

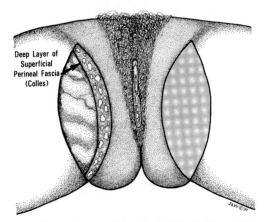

Fig. 1. Anatomic drawing of Colles' Fascia (*From* Lockwood TE. Fascial anchoring technique in medial thigh lifts. Plast Reconstr Surg 1988;82(2):299–304; with permission.)

distinct layers of adipose tissue. Between these two layers is a poorly defined superficial fascial layer.

The deep layer of the superficial perineal fascia as described by Lockwood is a distinct connective tissue layer lying below the subcutaneous fat of the perineum. The layer attaches to the ischiopubic rami of the bony pelvis, while anteriorly the layer is contiguous over the pubis with Scarpa's fascia of the abdominal wall. Posteriorly, the layer fuses with the posterior border of the urogenital diaphragm. At the junction of the perineum and medial thigh, a dense area of this strong Colles' fascia can be identified. Colles' fascia provides the anatomic shelf that defines the perineal thigh crease.

One can identify the Colles' fascia by, first, dissecting to the origin of the adductor muscles on the ischiopubic ramus and then retracting the skin and superficial fat of the vulva medially. The Colles' fascial roll lies at the deepest and most lateral aspect of the vulvar soft tissue.

The femoral triangle should be identified and preserved to reduce the chance for complications because deep dissection can lead to disruption of the lymphatic channels. Damage to these important structures can result in prolonged edema and even lymphatic collections.

Patient selection

One of the earliest signs of aging of the lower extremities is the presentation of medial thigh laxity. The skin of the superior medial thigh is quite thin, which may allow for the development of early ptosis. Women begin to present with these symptoms between the ages of 35 and 45. They also commonly complain of fat deposition in the trochanteric and hip areas as well as in the medial thigh. It is important to address the lower torso

circumferentially with suction lipectomy at the time of medial thigh lift.

Two factors need to be addressed to ensure a long-lasting and effective medial thigh lift. On physical exam, the degree of skin laxity and lipodystrophy must be quantified. Once these factors are correctly analyzed, the patient can then be classified and an appropriate treatment plan can be determined.

The lower body lift typically addresses the lateral thigh. The fat is removed through liposuction and direct excision. The skin laxity is improved with a combination of excision and via the process of discontinuous undermining.

The medial thigh is addressed with the thighplasty. However, in the MWL patient, the thigh must be evaluated for the degree of skin laxity, the quality of skin, the degree of deflation, and the overall extent of deformity. These factors are more pronounced in the MWL patient then in the classic medial thighplasty patient. Therefore, we have found that the classic approach to thigh lift does not address all of the anatomic problems found in the MWL patient. Over time, we have transitioned from the vertical vector Lockwood approach to a horizontal vector approach (Fig. 2).

Classification of medial thigh patients

There are two separate categories of medial thigh patients. They are divided into those patients who have undergone MWL and those that have not. The non-MWL patients are divided into four categories. Patients who present with type I medial thigh deformity and possess only lipodystrophy with no sign of skin laxity can be treated with liposuction alone (Fig. 3). Those patients who present with skin laxity confined to the upper one-third of the thigh require liposuction and a horizontally orientated skin excision (Fig. 4). The horizontal excision is only to correct the vertical laxity of the proximal 1/3 medial thigh. In general, as the degree of skin laxity progresses from the upper and medial to the entire medial thigh, the size of the vertical skin resection increases.

Finally, the advent and success of morbid obesity surgery has led to an increasing number of patients with significant medial thigh laxity after MWL. We place these patients in a separate category. There are two types of patients after MWL. The type I MWL are those patients that demonstrate skin laxity over the entire thigh but do not demonstrate significant residual lipodystrophy (often denoted as deflated) (Fig. 5). These patients are treated with a horizontal vector thigh lift. Patients who demonstrate both skin laxity and significant lipodystrophy (denoted as nondeflated) benefit from a staged procedure (Fig. 6). The suction lipectomy can be

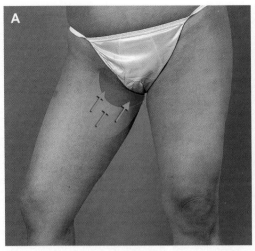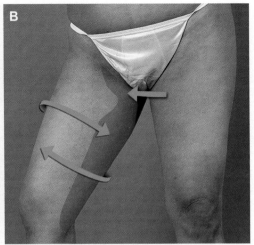

Fig. 2. (*A*) Classic Lockwood medial thighplasty. (*B*) Vertical incision thighplasty. (Green shading indicates liposuction. Orange shading indicates resection. Arrows indicate vectors of pull.)

Surgical technique

Classic medial thigh lift

In the classic medial thigh lift, the patient is marked in the standing anterior position with the knees

performed at the first stage combined with a lower body lift. This is followed by a second-stage, horizontally based medial thigh lift operation 3 to 6 months later to achieve an aesthetic thigh.

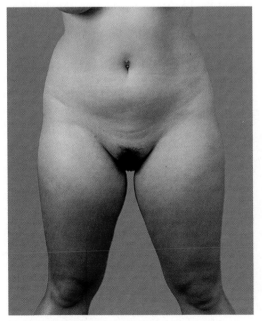

Fig. 3. Candidate for medial thigh liposuction.

apart. In this position, retraction of the skin both medially and posteriorly demonstrates the amount of skin to be removed. In addition, the location of fat deposits are delineated and marked for liposuction. The femoral triangles are marked to avoid dissection into the lymphatics. The incision is marked from the level of the ischium along the inner surface of the buttock's fold medially and inferiorly to the labia majora. The location of the incisions and the need to add a vertical component are determined by the classification of the thigh laxity. In general, if the skin laxity extends beyond the upper one-third of the thigh, then a vertical component is needed to contour the thigh. The range of excision of redundant tissue is estimated, usually between 4 and 8 cm, and an inferior proposed line of excision is marked to complete the potential ellipse to be excised.

When additional body contouring is performed, the patient is first placed in the prone position. This allows for both hip and lateral thigh liposuction. Once completed, the patient is placed in the supine position and the legs are circumferentially prepped from the hips down to below the knees. Further liposuction is performed as necessary. Once this is complete, the medial thigh is addressed and the legs are placed in the frog-leg position. We use foot compression devices for deep venous thrombosis prophylaxis in every case.

The more proximal incision is then made. Superficial dissection is imperative to preserve lymphatics around the femoral triangle. This area is then undermined down to the caudal incision. Once this mark is confirmed, the skin is then resected. The Colles' fascia is then identified. This structure

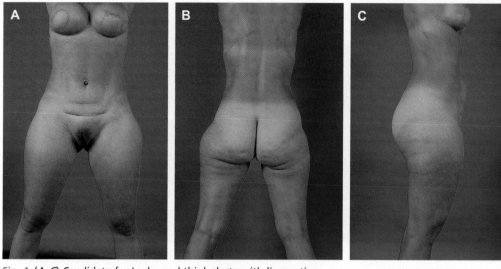

Fig. 4. (A–C) Candidate for Lockwood thighplasty with liposuction.

is best identified with traction applied on the lateral aspect of the fascia. Digital dissection using a dry gauze sponge most readily preserves the Colles' fascia. It is also important to limit undermining to the superficial level. The surgeon must preserve the soft-tissue bundle coursing between the mons pubis and femoral triangle. This soft-tissue bundle appears to reduce the risk of lymphatic complications. Anchoring sutures, 2-0 polydioxanone, are placed to incorporate Colles' fascia with the subdermal layer of both superior and inferior skin flaps. These sutures can be permanent. However, we favor large absorbable sutures. The deep dermal sutures are placed with 3-0 polydioxanone and 4-0 Monocryl subcuticular suture. Finally, Dermabond is used to seal the skin closure. Small drains (10F catheter) are usually placed before the closure of the skin. Compression garments are not used for 2 weeks, giving the incision time to heal. Early compression often leads to moisture and wound breakdown.

In the postoperative period, the patient is out of bed and ambulating the night of surgery. The drains are placed to wall suction for 24 hours and then to bulb suction. All patients receive perioperative antibiotics (Ancef) and a morphine patient-controlled analgesia pump. The majority of patients are discharged the day following surgery. The drains are

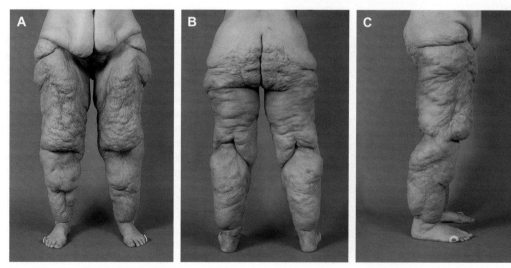

Fig. 5. (A–C) Deflated MWL patient.

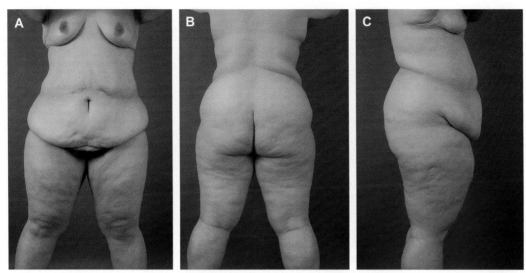

Fig. 6. (*A–C*) Nondeflated MWL patient.

removed in the office once the drain output is less than 30 mL (Figs. 7 and 8).

Medial thigh lift for massive weight loss patients

The change in design addresses the unique laxity of the medial thigh in the MWL patient. The classic technique described above has its vector of pull vertically toward the groin. Much of the morbidity, such as recurrent ptosis and traction deformity of the labia, appears to be related to this pull. In the MWL patient, this risk is increased as greater demands are placed in an effort to raise more of the distal thigh. The horizontal laxity seen in the MWL patient is often quite severe and difficult to completely address with the classic vertical pull (Fig. 9). The classic vertical pull also cannot address the middle distal third of the leg.

The vertical medial thigh lift uses both an anterior and posterior horizontal vector to accomplish thigh contouring. It does not rely on any type of vertical elevation or pull. All of the tension is focused along the medial aspect of the thigh, closing the thigh as a cylinder. The horizontal incision is limited to removal of the "dog ear" and does not contribute to the actual lift of the medial thigh. There is no need for tension closure to the Colles' as the tension is distributed along the cylinderic medial thigh closure from the knee to the groin.

Preoperative marking

The patient is marked in the standing position with the legs slightly apart. To eliminate lost time in the preoperative holding area, we now mark the patient in the office the day before surgery.

This allows for adequate time to mark the patient in a deliberate unhurried manner. It also allows for time to further educate the patient as to the location of the incision and placement of drains. Standardized photography is performed to accurately record the markings.

The first step is to outline the areas of lipodystrophy around the knee and lower one-third of the thigh. This enables the surgeon to taper the lower thigh with liposuction when necessary. Next, the desired ultimate location of the medial thigh incision is marked from the lower aspect of the knee to the groin crease (Fig. 10). The skin is then transposed from the anterior thigh toward the posterior thigh to meet this previously drawn line. This serves to delineate the amount of skin to be resected. The same technique is done from the posterior thigh toward the anterior thigh to determine the extent of resection of the posterior thigh. This should lead to a wedgelike resection. Once these marks are in place, the final incision lines are drawn. The anterior incision is drawn such that a "bottleneck" area of skin is preserved more proximally. Skin posterior and proximally is more adherent and less mobile. The bottleneck accounts for this and helps prevent anterior migration of the scar and visibility. The bottleneck helps keep the incision more hidden in the groin crease and more effectively addresses the less mobile proximal, posterior thigh. The posterior line, however, follows the line determined during the initial transposition of the skin. This design allows the thigh to be closed as a cylinder without any tension on the groin. There is no need to anchor the flaps to the Colles'

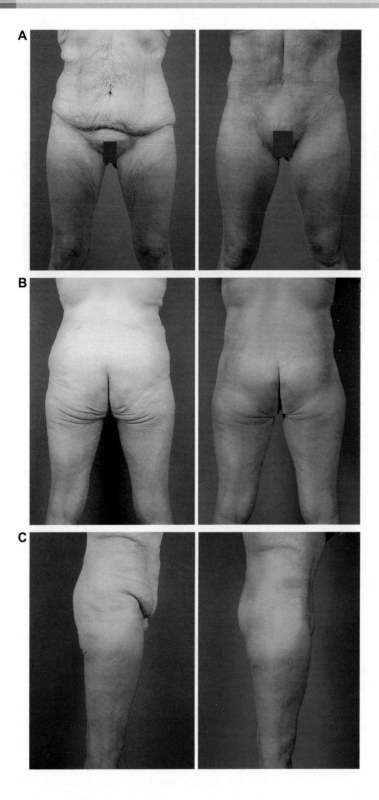

Fig. 7. (*A–C*) Deflated MWL patient. Before procedure (*left*). One-year following lower body lift with autologous gluteal augmentation and Lockwood thighplasty (*right*).

fascia. In addition, this technique eliminates the need for the prone position and avoids an incision in the buttock crease as the posterior laxity is rotated forward and excised.

Patient positioning

The patient is positioned on the operating room table in the supine position. We have found that the use of spreader bars to hold the legs abducted

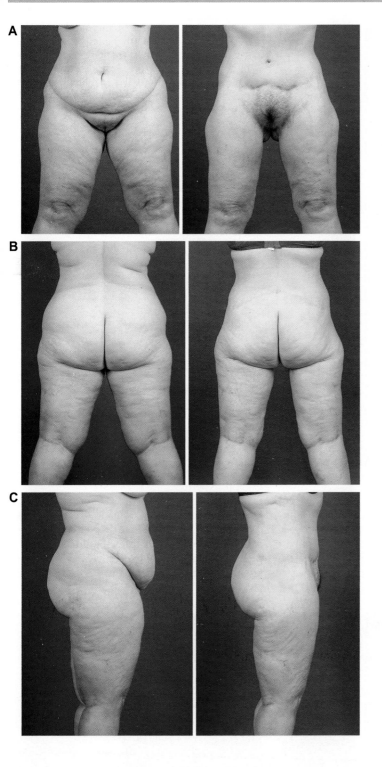

Fig. 8. (*A–C*) Preoperative (*left*) and 3-year status postabdominoplasty liposuction of thighs and Lockwood thighplasty (*right*).

allows the surgeon to sit between the legs (Fig. 11). This can reduce some of the neck strain associated with this operation. The patient should have sequential compression devices and a Foley catheter placed. All pressure points should be well padded to protect the patient.

Operative technique

As in the classic technique, the thigh is first addressed with ultrasound-assisted liposuction. In those patients that are MWL but are nondeflated, we use a two-stage approach. Aggressive liposuction is done at the time of the body lift. The resection is

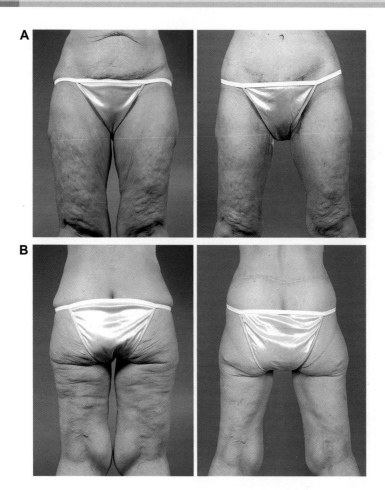

Fig. 9. (*A* and *B*) Lockwood medial thighplasty on deflated MWL patient. Preoperation (*left*). Postoperation (*right*). Note lack of improvement in distal third of thigh and knee.

done at a second stage, preferably 6 months later. In those patients that have lost much of the deep subcutaneous layer, the two procedures can be performed at the same operation. However, the use of liposuction is usually limited to the area around the knee.

The anterior incision is made first and carried down toward the level of the deep fascia. To ensure lymphatic preservation, care should be taken to preserve the greater saphenous vein as well as the fat around and deep to the vessel. Often the

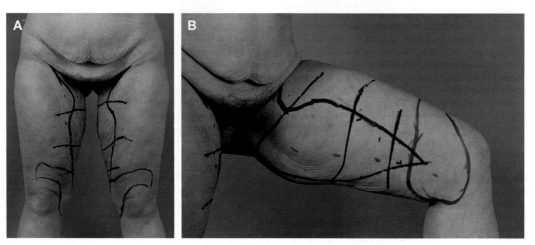

Fig. 10. (*A* and *B*) Preoperative marking of vertical thighplasty.

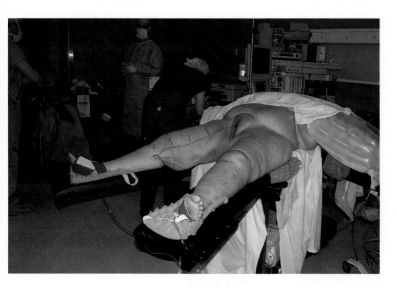

very low*Fig. 11.* Positioning using spreader bars.

posterior branch of the saphenous vein is ligated. At times it is necessary to divide some of the side branches of the saphenous vein to the flap. This can be quickly accomplished using an automatic surgical clip applier. If the patient has undergone previous liposuction, as is often performed as a first stage in the nondeflated MWL patient, a scar plane can often be identified and followed. The dissection is then carried to the posterior marks. Skin to be resected is then confirmed. Careful hemostasis is obtained and a 15F-catheter drain is placed through a separate stab incision. Excision of the skin commences distally to proximally. The anterior incision line is mobilized posteriorly to confirm the posterior extent of resection. This proceeds proximally and the tissue is removed. The two flaps are temporarily closed with staples. The wound is then closed in layers. The superficial fascial system is closed with a running #0 polydioxanone suture. The running sutures allow for even distribution of tension and minimizes the problem of suture extrusion of the knots. The deep dermis is then closed with interrupted 2-0 polydioxanone and 3-0 Monocryl sutures. The epidermis is closed with a running 3-0 Monocryl suture.

The postoperative care is similar to that for the classic medial thigh lift as described above. However, the use of Dermabond to seal the wound minimizes the need for any complex surgical dressing. We have also abandoned any use of Ace wraps or other constricting garments around the medial thigh for at least 2 weeks. In the past, we used a two-layer running closure of the dermis. While this speeds up the time of closure, it can be problematic if the patient has wound-healing problems. Localized wound-healing problems can be

propagated with the disruption of the sutures (Figs. 12–14).

Discussion

Most of the recent techniques of medial thigh lift are now based on Lockwood's concept of supporting the thigh lift with sutures to create a superficial fascialike suspension [11]. The techniques all attempt to anchor the lift on some portion of Colles' fascia. This technique of closure appears to address many of the problems associated with the original techniques of the medial thigh lift. The recent modifications all attempt to increase the fascial support and decrease tension on the healing scars. No studies have examined the superiority of one technique over another. However, there is clearly merit in limiting the size of the tissue flaps and the degree of undermining. The need for more aggressive techniques to support the flap do not appear to reduce the complications and may actually lead to other complications, such as seroma or contour deformity of the mons pubis.

The Lockwood medial thigh lift can be employed when treating the non-MWL patients. However, we have found that this technique does not address many of the anatomic issues encountered in the MWL patient or the entire aging thigh. The technique described minimizes the horizontal incision and the need for vertical lift. It instead relies on a vertical incision and horizontal pull. The groin incision is limited to remove the "dog ear" and there is no need for tension closure to Colles' fascia. This technique also avoids the T incision. The more recent addition of the "bucket handle" to the anterior incision has further refined the

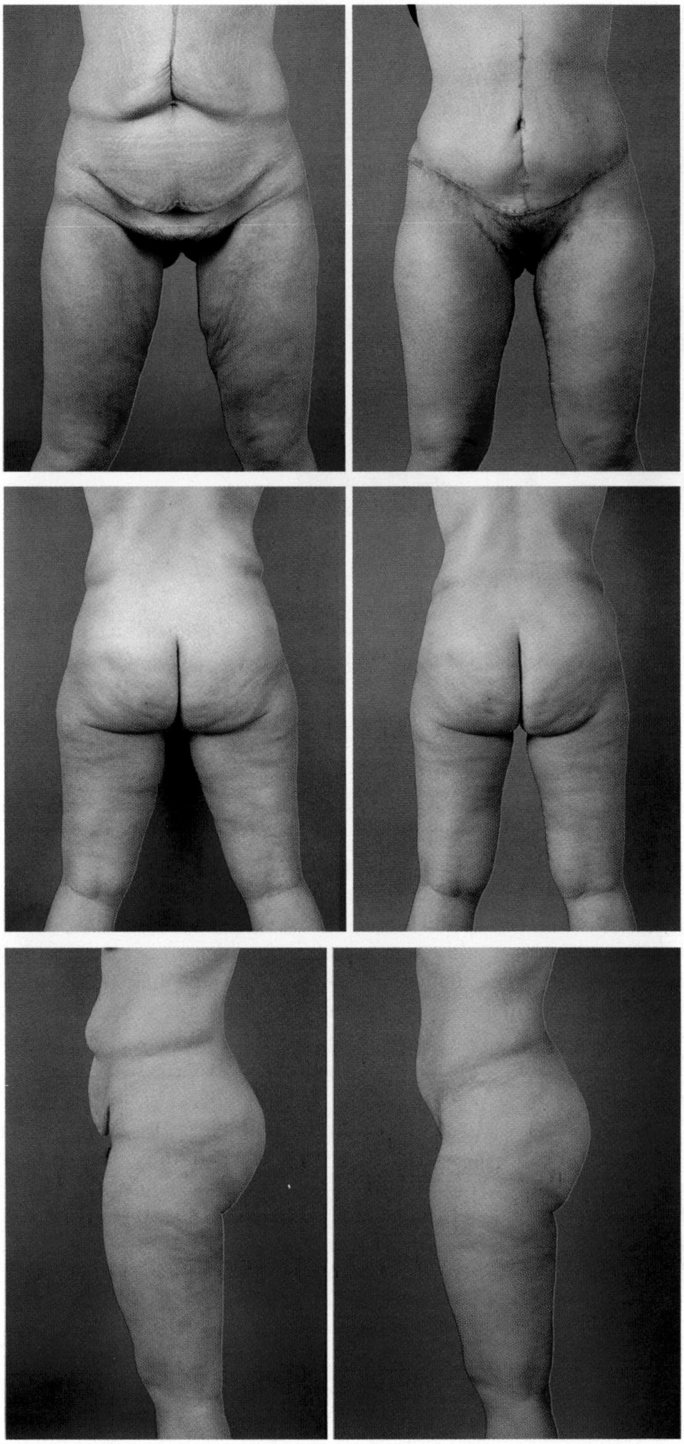

Fig. 12. (A–C) Before (left) and 6 months after (right) abdominoplasty and vertical thigh lift.

closure of the medial thigh. This has led to a more concealed incision and less undermining of the anterior aspect of the groin. We have also begun to explore the use of an additional suprapatellar incision on those patients with significant excess skin over the knee.

The critical determinant of success in this procedure is in the preoperative assessment and surgical

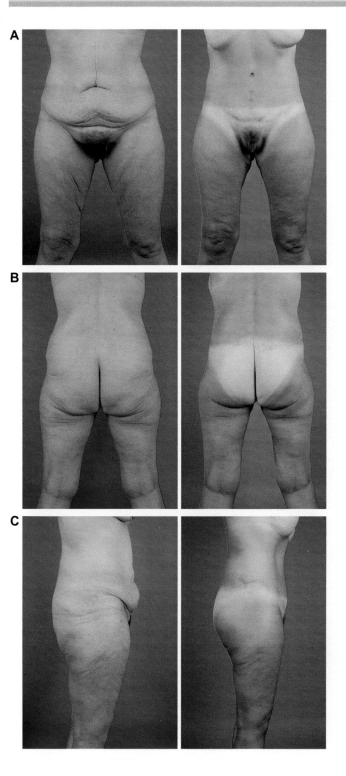

Fig. 13. (*A–C*) Before procedures (*left*). Eighteen months after lower body lift with autologous gluteal augmentation and 8 months after vertical thighplasty (*right*).

planning. The operation can then be tailored to the patient's individual needs based on the preoperative assessment of the amount of skin laxity as well as on the location of the lipodystrophy. The use of the thigh classification system simplifies this process and allows the surgeon to compare patient results based on a standardized classification. A thigh lift design based on the correct

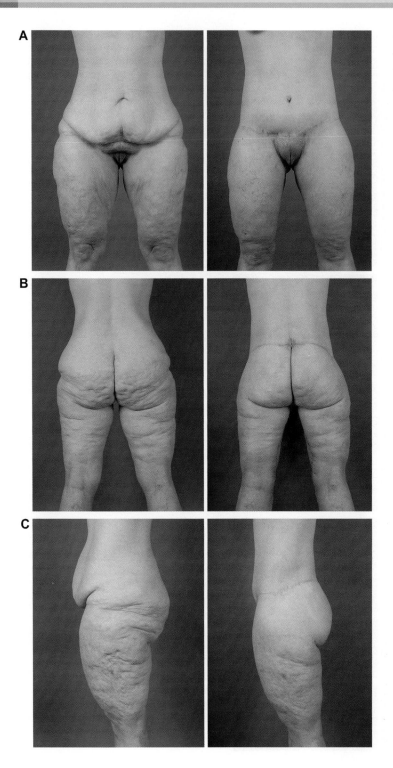

Fig. 14. (*A–C*) Before procedures (*left*). Nine months after lower body lift and 6 months after vertical thighplasty (*right*).

medial thigh classification should lead to an operation that best suits the patient's anatomic needs and results in a cosmetically acceptable thighplasty.

References

[1] Lewis JR Jr. Correction of ptosis of the thighs: the thigh lift. Plast Reconstr Surg 1966;37(6):494–8.

[2] Lockwood TE. Fascial anchoring technique in medial thigh lifts. Plast Reconstr Surg 1988; 82(2):299–304.

[3] Lockwood T. Lower body lift with superficial fascial system suspension. Plast Reconstr Surg 1993; 92(6):1112–22 [discussion: 1123–5].

[4] Candiani P, Campiglio GL, Signorini M. Fascio-fascial suspension technique in medial thigh lifts. Aesthetic Plast Surg 1995;19(2): 137–40.

[5] Spirito D. Medial thigh lift and DE.C.LI.VE. Aesthetic Plast Surg 1998;22(4):298–300.

[6] Ersek RA, Salisbury AV. The saddle lift for tight thighs. Aesthetic Plast Surg 1995;19(4):341–3.

[7] Pitanguy IP. Surgical reduction of the abdomen, thighs and buttocks. Surg Clin North Am 1971; 51(2):479–89.

[8] Planas J. The "Crural Meloplasty" for lifting of the thighs. Clin Plast Surg 1975;2:495–503.

[9] Le Louarn C, Pascal JF. The concentric medial thigh lift. Aesthetic Plast Surg 2004;28(1):20–3 [Epub 2004 Mar 25].

[10] Vilain R, Dardour JC. Aesthetic surgery of the medial thigh. Ann Plast Surg 1986;17(3): 176–83.

[11] Hurwitz DJ. Single-staged total body lift after massive weight loss. Ann Plast Surg 2004;52(5): 435–41.

CLINICS IN
PLASTIC
SURGERY

Clin Plastic Surg 35 (2008) 165–172

Thigh Reduction in the Massive Weight Loss Patient

Albert Cram, MD, FACS, Al Aly, MD, FACS*

- Patient presentation
- Preoperative evaluation
- Surgical technique
- Markings
- Postoperative care

- Results
- Complications
- Summary
- References

With the variety of bariatric procedures available today, there is a steadily growing stream of massive weight loss patients. Although there have been major advances in upper extremity and upper and lower truncal contouring, the lower extremity often remains the most difficult to treat. Historically, thigh reductions were designed to treat minor medial thigh laxity. As a response to some of the difficulties that can be encountered in medial thigh lifting, Lockwood [1,2] developed a technique designed to prevent migration of the horizontal perineal scar and labial spreading in the female patient. Although this technique is useful in treating the ordinary minor medial thigh laxity, it is generally not effective for the massive weight loss patient deformity. The technique described in this article is specifically designed for the massive weight loss patient who presents with extensive thigh deformity. For lesser deformities more traditional techniques should be used.

Two basic principles are very useful to understand and use in plastic surgery. First, it is important for a plastic surgeon to understand normal anatomy of any structure that they plan to reconstruct. The overall anatomy of the thigh is similar to a cone with a hard inner core, the musculoskeletal system, and an outer cover made up of the skin-fat envelope.

The skin-fat envelope is more adherently attached to the musculoskeletal inner core on the outer half of the cone. The top of the cone is located at the perineal crease and the bottom at the knee. Unlike a cone, however, the widest aspect of the cone is located 2 to 3 in below the top of the cone, and the narrowest is usually located 2 to 3 in above the knee.

The second basic principle that is imperative for plastic surgeons is to define the deformity that is encountered. The entire thigh skin-fat envelope descends inferiorly with the process of weight gain and loss. It seems that most of the excess that occurs after massive weight loss is vertical in nature. Careful examination, however, reveals that the skin-fat envelope is less tightly adherent medially than laterally. Although there is a certain degree of vertical excess in these thighs, most of the excess is horizontal in nature, and because the medial adherence is not strong, the tissues in this area descend giving the impression that it is vertical rather than horizontal excess that presents (Fig. 1).

Based on this understanding of the deformity, the authors developed a vertical resection to deal with the medial horizontal excess in the thighs of massive weight loss patients. This technique is used after a belt lipectomy is initially performed, in a separate procedure. This lifts the lateral aspect of the

Iowa City Plastic Surgery, 501 12th Avenue, Suite 102, Coralville, IA 52241, USA
* Corresponding author.
E-mail address: mdplastic@aol.com (A. Aly).

doi:10.1016/j.cps.2007.09.005

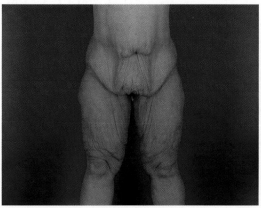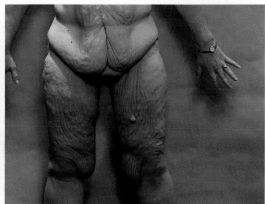

Fig. 1. Two massive weight loss patients demonstrating how the skin-fat envelope drapes over the underlying musculoskeletal core. Note the skin-fat envelope is more attached anteriorly and laterally than medially, leading to medial vertical descent of the mostly horizontal excess.

cone, and depending on the translation of pull that the particular patient's tissues allow, the belt lipectomy also lifts the anterior and posterior thigh.

The surgeon must also keep in mind the superficial vascular branches present in the leg, and most importantly the lymphatic structures and their location. The saphenous vein and its largest branches are subject to possible injury during many of the procedures useful in thigh contouring. Many of these patients have significant varicose vein problems and in appropriate cases the saphenous vein or segments of it may be excised during a medial skin resection. The lymphatic drainage of the leg is primarily concentrated medially, but the vessels tend to lie deeper than the saphenous vein until the vessels begin to coalesce in the femoral triangle where the saphenous vein turns to join the femoral vein. Injury to the lymphatic drainage of the leg can result in the disastrous complication of disabling lower-extremity lymphedema, which is usually permanent and which often results in medicolegal actions. The operations chosen for thigh recontouring should be designed to avoid this complication at all costs.

excellent deflation of the fat and primarily a loose circumferential skin-fat envelope. These patients are ideal to operate on, but only after they have undergone a belt lipectomy to lift the anterior, lateral, and posterior thigh.

These first two types of presenting deformity are all too infrequent in the authors' practice. The most common thigh presentation in most female patients is one of a minimally deflated thigh despite an overall excellent weight loss and highly significant body mass index change. These patients most often undergo extensive liposuction of the thighs when their belt lipectomy is performed to deflate the thighs in preparation for an excisional procedure. In some patients that posses a very large amount of excess fat in the thighs, a number of preliminary liposuction procedures should be performed before the final liposuction procedure performed in conjunction with the belt lipectomy. Overall, to attain a significant improvement in the thighs, they should be deflated either naturally by the process of massive weight loss, or surgically by liposuction before their final excisional procedure.

Patient presentation

The type and extent of deformity seen in the thigh of the massive weight loss patient is extremely variable. Some patients never deposited much of their excess fat in their thigh region and may not require more than the belt lipectomy alone to achieve an acceptable contour. This is seen much more frequently in the male patient, but may also be seen in some females who have a genetic tendency to an "apple" fat storage configuration rather than a "pear" configuration.

Some patients who did deposit a high percentage of their excess fat in the thigh may come in with

Preoperative evaluation

During the initial evaluation of all massive weight loss patients a complete history and physical evaluation is essential. A thorough evaluation of the lower extremities should be carried out. Full body photographs should be done with a technique that allows good views from anterior, posterior, lateral, and oblique angles. Study of these photographs often reveals subtle asymmetries and helps to guide the operative plan in directions that were not always apparent on direct examination in the clinic. Specific to the lower extremity is a careful examination to rule out deep vein problems and to ensure that the patient does not have any pre-existing lymphedema. Significant venous problems should instigate a vascular consult, and any evidence of lymphedema should be considered a contraindication to lower-extremity recontouring.

Evaluation of the soft tissue excess should include an assessment of the horizontal and the vertical excess, its location, and the elasticity of the skin. The remaining lipodystrophy should be ascertained in all the different regions of the thigh. The patient is asked to take the skin just above the inguinal ligament and pull upward, and the translation of pull is noted by how far down the lateral and anterior thigh the effect extends.

It is very important for those who are going to include a horizontal resection of skin to evaluate the degree to which any downward traction is transmitted across the perineal junction to produce lateral traction on the labia. The complication of labial spread with subsequent exposure of the labia minor can produce significant symptoms and has often been the primary complaint leading to medicolegal action in thigh-reduction procedures. The authors recommend avoiding horizontal excisions if at all possible, and where they must be done, extreme measures to prevent labial distraction are warranted, but occasionally unsuccessful.

Surgical technique

Overall, the technique discussed here creates a vertical wedge of tissue that is located on the medial aspect of the thigh. The vertical wedge is situated posteriorly enough so that if a horizontal component is needed to eliminate vertical excess, it does not cause distortion of the labia. The excision is also designed to reduce the risk of permanent lymphedema.

Markings

The markings are performed in the clinic, 1 to 2 days before surgery. The patient is placed first in the lithotomy position and the perineal crease as it extends into the infrabuttocks crease. Next, a point along that line, which ends up being the top of the ellipse, is marked. To determine this point, tissue is pinched along different points of the perineal crease, starting anteriorly and moving posteriorly. At some point the pinch has minimal effect on the position of the labia and that point is chosen and marked (Fig. 2).

With the patient standing and the knees approximately 10 to 12 in apart, a vertical line is drawn down the medial aspect of the thigh starting at the mark made on the perineal crease. This line is the center of a marked ellipse and estimates the

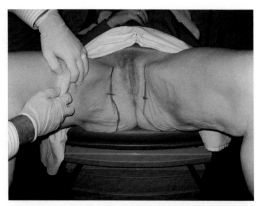

Fig. 2. The point along the perineal crease where there is minimal to no effect on labial position, should a horizontal component need to be used.

eventual position of the scar. Next, the double ellipse technique of marking, described in the authors' article on brachioplasty elsewhere in this issue, is used to mark the thighs. It is important to remember that the widest aspect of the normal thigh cone occurs 2 to 3 in below the perineal crease; the ellipse needs to be adjusted accordingly. Not having to make that area significantly narrow allows the ellipse to be fairly narrow near the top and helps reduce the need for a horizontal resection. In some patients, this incision has to extend all the way to the lowest point of knee excess, occasionally even dropping below the medial condyle. Horizontal hash marks are then made as guides about every 8 to 10 cm down the length of the ellipse as rough guides for reapproximation at the time of closure. In the operating room the patient is placed in the lithotomy position (Fig. 3).

The authors have tried a number of positions to perform thigh-reduction surgery and found that the lithotomy position is the most comfortable

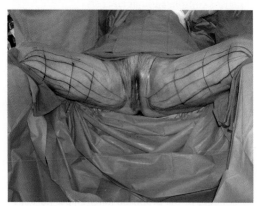

Fig. 3. Patient in the lithotomy position in the operating room.

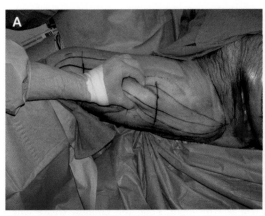
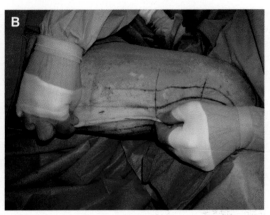

Fig. 4. Proposed area of resection before liposuction (*A*) and after liposuction (*B*). Note the remaining skin is essentially "paper thin."

and gives the greatest access to the areas involved. The soft tissues deep to the proposed inner ellipse, earmarked for resection, are then tumesced with liposuction fluid. This area is then aggressively liposuctioned, even suctioning the underside of the skin, to deflate completely the area of fat (Fig. 4).

This maneuver has two excellent benefits. First, liposuction eliminates the fat without injuring the lymphatics. This, along with avoiding injury to the femoral triangle with its very rich lymphatics, should greatly reduce or eliminate the risk of permanent lymphedema. Second, after liposuction, tailor tacking the edges of the inner ellipse with staples allows the surgeon both to visualize the final result and to adjust the markings before making any skin cuts. After the liposuction is completed, the inner ellipse edges are stapled together (Fig. 5).

If there are areas where the proposed resection is too tight or too loose, the line of resection can be adjusted appropriately. The staples are then removed, and the resection is performed using the segmental resection closure technique described in the previously mentioned brachioplasty article elsewhere in this issue. During the resection of tissue from one hash mark to the next, the skin is essentially peeled off of the underlying structures. No attempt is made to resect the deeper tissues unless they were to cause minor irregularities. The segmental resection closure technique allows the surgeon to excise tissue and close efficiently and quickly to prevent intraoperative edema from occurring. Initially, the temporary closure using this technique is performed with staples (Fig. 6).

The staples are then replaced with a two-layer closure and skin glue to cover the skin. At the superior end of the closure, because it is an area that has a high predilection for wound healing problems, the closure is reinforced with a few skin

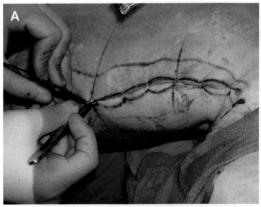
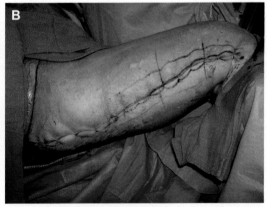

Fig. 5. Edges of the proposed inner ellipse partially approximated with staples (*A*) and after completion of the tailor tacking (*B*). This gives the surgeon the ability essentially to see the final result before committing to any surgical cuts.

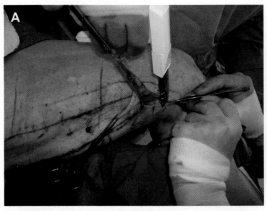
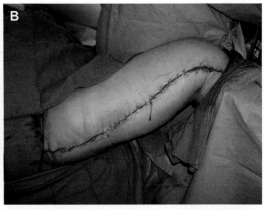

Fig. 6. Segmental resection closure technique. (*A*) The tissues are resected from one hash mark to the other and that segment is immediately stapled. (*B*) The temporary closure after the entire ellipse is resected.

staples that are kept in place for 2 to 3 weeks postoperatively.

"Dog ears" can potentially occur at the superior end of the closure. One way to prevent this from occurring is during the marking process where the width of the superior ellipse width is kept to a minimum based on the fact that the greatest width of the thigh operated on should be located 2 to 3 in below the perineal crease. Occasionally, however, the patient's anatomy dictates the necessity of a superior dog ear. The authors' solution to this problem is to extend the incision posteriorly, avoid extending anteriorly, and end up with the incision along the infrabuttocks crease (Fig. 7).

Postoperative care

At the end of the procedure the patient is placed in a tight liposuction-type garment. Most patients are admitted overnight for observation, although the procedure can be performed on an outpatient basis. The authors sometimes use closed suction drains, but more and more tend to go without drains. The patient is instructed on leg elevation and avoidance of lower-extremity dependency, especially standing and sitting with legs dependent, for months after surgery. If the patient tends to swell distally, the garment used needs to start at foot level and go up to the waist. They are also instructed to raise their legs twice a day to a level much higher than their waist and to massage the swelling from distal to proximal followed by application of the garment. It may take some patients up to 6 months not to swell when their legs are dependent. The superior skin staples are left in place for 2 to 3 weeks after surgery.

Results

The thigh-reduction technique presented here is designed to avoid labial spreading or scar migration

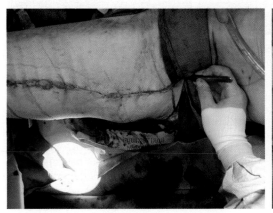
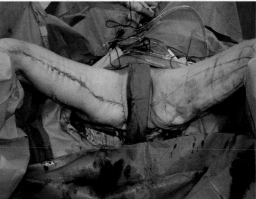

Fig. 7. Superior "dog ear" is handled. The vertical incision is extended posteriorly along the infrabuttocks crease, and the excess tissue is tailored.

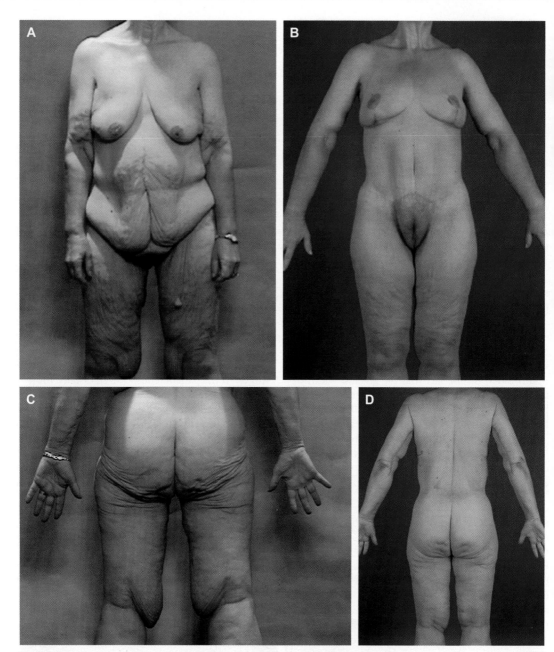

Fig. 8. Patient's photographs pre–belt lipectomy and thigh reduction (*A, C*) and approximately 2 years post– belt lipectomy and thigh reduction (*B, D*). She did not require further deflation before her thigh reduction.

issues encountered with perineal scars, and reduce the risk of lymphedema. It may not produce as much reduction and tightness in the upper third of the thigh, compared with other techniques that use a horizontal component, but it can produce some remarkable results in most patients (Figs. 8 and 9).

The authors almost never combine a belt lipectomy with a thigh lift in a single procedure because in some patients, especially those with extensive translation of pull, the effects on the medial thighs may be enough to eliminate the need for a thigh reduction all together. In most other patients, the improvement in the thighs reduces the extent of the thigh-reduction surgery, so it does not make sense to combine both in the same sitting and potentially end up doing more surgery than is needed if the thigh reduction is delayed.

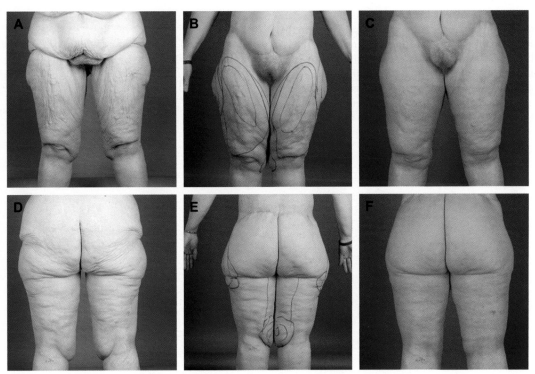

Fig. 9. (*A, D*) Patient whose thighs were still very inflated after she stabilized her weight loss. (*B, E*) After a belt lipectomy with concomitant liposuction of the thighs her thighs were still inflated. She underwent a secondary liposuction of the thighs and 6 months later underwent a thigh reduction procedure as described in this article. (*C, F*) Final result 2.5 years after initial procedure and after gaining some weight back.

Complications

Other than the common universal potential complications of bleeding, infection, and bad scarring, the most common complication encountered after thigh reduction, in the authors' patient population, is small areas of wound separation accompanied by delayed healing. The most likely place for this to occur is at the top of the closure, although areas anywhere along the incision can separate. In most instances these separations are relatively superficial and do not constitute a true dehiscence. Treatment usually involves conservative wound care and allowing these areas to heal by secondary intention.

Seromas can occur and they tend to be at the inferior end of the incision. It is interesting that since adopting the technique of leaving behind as much lymphatics as possible, the seroma rate has come down, although it is not zero. The authors do not believe that drains are needed in most of these patients and often do not use them. If seromas do occur they serially aspirate them and should they persist they are injected with a sclerosing agent, such as dicloxacillin or povidone-iodine. If the seroma still persists, then a small area of the incision is opened and the seroma cavity is exteriorized by placing a Penrose

drain through it and lightly wrapping the extremity until the seroma essentially "burns" itself out.

Labial spreading is a dreaded complication and the authors simply avoid using techniques that can potentially cause this complication. With the technique described in this article, it is extremely unlikely for this complication to develop.

All patients develop temporary distal extremity edema of varying degrees after vertical thigh reduction. The postoperative regimen described previously helps most patients regain their ability to clear edema within a few months. The technique itself helps preserve as many lymphatic channels as possible and avoids the major lymphatic drainage station of the lower extremity located in the femoral region. If permanent lymphedema should occur, its treatment is similar to the treatment of any patient with that process.

Summary

Thigh reduction after massive weight loss is a difficult operation with potential for significant complications. Understanding the normal anatomy and how the deformities develop after massive weight loss led to the design an operation that eliminates horizontal excess by resecting a vertical ellipse. The technique avoids the issue of labial spreading in the female patient by not putting any tension on the labia. It also avoids permanent lymphedema by leaving behind as many lymphatic channels as possible and avoiding operating on the femoral triangle area. Since adoption of this technique thigh reductions have become less stressful.

References

[1] Lockwood T. Superficial fascial system (SFS) of the trunk and extremities: a new concept. Plast Reconstr Surg 1991;87:1009–18.

[2] Lockwood TE. Lower body lift and medial thigh lift. In: Aly AS, editor. Body contouring after massive weight loss. St Louis (MO): Quality Medical Publishing; 2005. p. 148–81.

ELSEVIER
SAUNDERS

CLINICS IN
PLASTIC
SURGERY

Clin Plastic Surg 35 (2008) 173–183

Safety First: Precautions for the Massive Weight Loss Patient

Steven P. Davison, MD, DDS, FACS*, Mark W. Clemens, MD

- Preoperative precautions
  Medical status
  Nutritional deficiencies
  Diabetes
- Peri- and intraoperative precautions
  *Antibiotic prophylaxis and infection
     control*
  Anesthesia evaluation
  Positioning

  Case three
  Hypothermia
  Incisional closure
- Postoperative precautions
  *Deep vein thrombosis and pulmonary
     embolism prophylaxis*
- Summary
- References

Bariatric surgery has led to success in maintaining long-term weight loss and has become one of the best surgical options for morbidly obese patients [1,2]. From 1998 to 2006, the number of bariatric procedures increased from 13,000 to just less than 200,000 [3]. This likely represents just the tip of the iceberg as it becomes more available to the potential 15 million Americans who are now classified as morbidly obese (defined as a body mass index [BMI]>40 kg/m² or BMI>35 kg/m² with a major comorbid condition). A recent announcement by Medicare to expand coverage of this procedure is expected to increase demand further. The upward trend in bariatric surgery has led to a concomitant increase in postgastric bypass body-contouring procedures [4]. Between 2000 and 2004, these procedures increased 77%, with approximately 106,000 body-contouring procedures performed in 2004 [5]. The number of patients who have experienced massive weight loss is on the increase, and this growing population has special needs that must be addressed adequately to ensure that procedures

are performed safely. Patient safety is the highest priority of the body-contouring surgeon (Box 1).

Two groups of patients settle out in this evolving spectrum of patients who have lost weight. One group is the thin patient trapped in the sac of excess skin, a patient who has had successful bariatric surgery. They are healthier than they were. The second group has lost weight, but body-contouring surgery, such as panniculectomy, is a step toward a healthier self. Their preexisting conditions add issues. We present three case vignettes to illustrate this distinction and their inherent risks and perioperative concerns.

Preoperative precautions

Medical status

Patient safety starts with an emphasis on preoperative planning and strategy. Special attention must be addressed to the current medical status of the patient who has lost a massive amount of weight. An extensive history includes recording the patient's

Department of Plastic Surgery, Georgetown University Medical Center, 3800 Reservoir Road NW, Washington DC, 20007, USA
* Corresponding author.
E-mail address: spd2@georgetown.edu (S.P. Davison).

doi:10.1016/j.cps.2007.08.002

> **Box 1: Summary of safety precautions for the patient who has lost a massive amount of weight**
>
> Addressing underlying medical conditions
> Nutritional status and supplementation
> Infection control
> Patient positioning
> Prevention of hypothermia
> Meticulous surgical technique for wound healing
> Deep vein thrombosis prophylaxis

maximal weight and BMI, type of surgery or method of weight loss, and current stable weight and BMI. The type of procedure performed has implications for what type of nutritional deficiencies may be encountered, as seen in the difference between specific vitamin and mineral deficiencies in malabsorptive versus restrictive bariatric surgery. The preoperative work-up should include a panel of laboratory tests at least 2 weeks before any planned procedure to allow for enough time to address and correct any deficiencies. Most body-contouring procedures are performed between 12 and 18 months after weight loss surgery, and a documented constant weight for at least 3 months helps to ensure weight stabilization. The bariatric group commonly has underlying hypertension, undiagnosed diabetes, and heart disease with such manifestations as atrial fibrillation. Any history of deep venous thrombosis should have been addressed adequately; if it is warranted, the patient should be anticoagulated properly. Given the complexity of various diseases and comorbidities affecting the patient who has lost massive amounts of weight, a thorough preoperative clearance and cardiac evaluation by an internist and an experienced anesthesiology team is preferable to help optimize his/her medical condition. The history should include questions regarding drug allergies, continued use of diet pills (eg, phentermine), herbal supplementation that may affect anesthesia, and any medications used to treat autoimmune diseases (eg, steroids) that may contribute to poor incisional healing. Phentermine and fenfluramine, in alternating circulating serotonin levels, have been linked to aortic valve injury and pulmonary hypertension. Consequently, many patients may demonstrate the potential adverse effects of valvular heart disease [6].

The presence of a regular exercise program is a positive sign that can indicate that a patient is taking steps to preserve one's lean BMI. Smoking significantly decreases local cutaneous flow, and it should be documented, addressed, and strongly discouraged with the patient. We advise having a detailed medical questionnaire specific to the patient who has lost a massive amount of weight (Fig. 1) [7].

Nutritional deficiencies

Often, the patient's original gastric bypass procedure will have contributed to significant malabsorption and protein deficiencies. In addition to routine laboratory tests, such as electrolyte analysis and a complete blood cell count with differential, patients who have lost a massive amount of weight will need to have their ferritin, folate, calcium, vitamin B_{12}, prealbumin, and albumin levels checked (Table 1) [8,9].

Long-term and acute nutritional status should be assessed (optimal albumin is >3.5 g/dL or total lymphocyte count >1500). Any detected deficiencies are corrected immediately to prevent incisional healing delays. Patients who are not regularly following up with their bariatric physician may signal a noncompliant patient or it may reflect a lack of appropriate postoperative care by the bariatric surgeon. Patients who have undergone gastric bypass rarely receive adequate dietary calcium without supplementation. In malabsorptive bypass procedures, the bowel does not readily absorb calcium, and the stomach is shortened drastically, resulting in less opportunity for calcium uptake. Twice-daily chewable calcium supplements along with a regular exercise program promote calcium build-up. Common vitamin-replacement regimens include a multivitamin, zinc, and protein. Absence of luminal intrinsic factor after gastric bypass surgery can lead to a diminished vitamin B_{12}. Decreased vitamin B_{12}, folate, or both were observed in 88% of patients who underwent jejunoileal bypass surgery for morbid obesity [10,11]. Therefore, all patients should be supplemented with vitamin B_{12} and folate, a key step to lowering blood levels of homocysteine, which has been linked to cardiovascular disease [9]. Patients who are deficient in thiamine (vitamin B_1) may exhibit signs of limb weakness, gait instability, and confusion. These symptoms are manifestations of Wernicke's encephalopathy, which may, although rare, progress to permanent neuropathies and coma, referred to as Korsakoff's syndrome.

During body-contouring procedures, large areas of well-vascularized excess skin excision can lead to excessive and significant blood loss that warrants adequately addressing a preoperative anemia and offering the banking of blood for a likely operative transfusion. Underlying anemia may be the result of deficiencies in folate and vitamin B_{12}, a consequence of gastric bypass procedures that use small stomach pouches. Chromagen Forte (Savage Laboratories, Melville, New York) is a common supplementation that is used for vitamin B_{12}, folate, and

MEDICAL QUESTIONNAIRE
FOR MASSIVE-WEIGHT-LOSS PATIENTS

Name _____ Date _____

How old are you?_____

How tall are you?_____

How much did you weigh at your greatest weight?_____

How much do you weigh now?_____ How long have you been that weight?_____

Do you have any of the following medical problems?

- Heart disease   No_____ Yes_____
- Lung disease   No_____ Yes_____
- High blood pressure   No_____ Yes_____
- Diabetes   No_____ Yes_____
- Intestinal problems   No_____ Yes_____
- Kidney or liver problems   No_____ Yes_____
- Ovary or uterine problems (If female)   No_____ Yes_____
- Bleeding disorders   No_____ Yes_____
- Thyroid disease   No_____ Yes_____
- History of depression, anxiety, or psychosis   No_____ Yes_____
- History of seizures   No_____ Yes_____

Do you smoke?   No_____ Yes_____

Do you drink a lot of alcohol?   No_____ Yes_____

Have you had any surgeries, especially abdominal surgeries?   No_____ Yes_____

Where are the scars?_____

Do you take any medicines regularly? Please list them.

_____   _____   _____
_____   _____   _____
_____   _____   _____
_____   _____   _____

Are you allergic to any medicines? Please list them.

_____   _____   _____
_____   _____   _____
_____   _____   _____
_____   _____   _____

Fig. 1. Questionnaire for the patient who has lost a massive amount of weight. (*From* Aly AS, editor. Body contouring after massive weight loss. St. Louis (MO): Quality Medical Publishing; 2006. p. 55; with permission.)

vitamin C. Some severe deficiencies may warrant vitamin B_{12} injections.

Case one

A 45-year-old woman with a BMI of 30 kg/m² and status postgastric banding presented for body-contouring surgery after an approximately 140-lb weight loss. Her requests included mastopexy with augmentation and a lower body lift. Preoperative evaluation showed that the patient's health concerns were now limited to a vitamin B_{12} deficiency for which she received subcutaneous injections every 12 hours. The patient was able to give directed blood donations and underwent uneventful

surgery. This patient represents the first group: post-bariatric surgery.

Diabetes

There is particular concern for underlying medical conditions related to morbid obesity, such as diabetes. Diabetic patients have a depressed immune response and, hence, have increased susceptibility to infection and are especially prone to *Streptococcus* and *Staphylococcus* skin infections. Diabetes and perioperative hyperglycemia were shown independently to increase the prevalence of surgical site infections (SSIs) [12–15]. A history of diabetes was shown to increase the risk for SSIs by as much as

Table 1: Preoperative laboratory tests

Test	Rationale
Total protein and albumin	3-wk nutrition marker
Prealbumin	3-d nutrition marker
Total lymphocyte count	Acute nutrition marker
Ferritin	Iron deficiency
Hemoglobin	Anemia
Calcium	Mineral deficiency
Vitamin B$_{12}$ and folate	Vitamin deficiency

2.7-fold. Similarly, the risk for SSIs and nosocomial infections correlates with the degree of glucose elevation [12]. Waiting until the diabetes is controlled may not be possible, and bariatric surgery may improve glucose tolerance.

We place patients on low-dose insulin sliding scales and Accu-checks with meals and at night. For patients with a demonstrated hemoglobin A1c of greater than 7%, low-carbohydrate meals and an insulin drip are initiated upon admission to the hospital for strict glycemic control. Daily management of glycemic control, which is burdensome and time consuming, has shown its efficacy in the short- and long-term prevention of morbidity [14,15]. The goals of intensive therapy should be preprandial glucose concentrations between 70 and 120 mg/dL and postprandial concentrations of less than 180 mg/dL. Any patients who have hemoglobin A1c greater than 6.05% or hyperglycemia during the perioperative period require appropriate follow-up with formal testing for diabetes.

Case 2 graphically illustrates the surgical risks in this patient group.

Case two

A 63-year-old woman lost 75 lbs to stabilize her BMI at 54.9 km/m^2. She had a medical history significant for breast cancer, diabetes, chronic obstructive pulmonary disease (COPD) on continuous oxygen, hypertension, lymphedema, and hypothyroidism. She presented with a significant amount of excess skin and large lymphadenomous sacs on the inner portion of both thighs. She was a smoker and had undergone a previous right mastectomy and panniculectomy. During her hospital course, she was placed on an insulin drip for control of diabetes. The leg masses were staged with partial closure and vacuum assisted closure (V.A.C., Kinetic Concepts, Inc., San Antonio, Texas) dressing application. Second-stage closure of the left thigh was performed with a concurrent ventral hernia repair performed by general surgery. The postoperative course resulted in an acute COPD exacerbation that

required a short ICU stay. She was followed as an outpatient by an infectious disease physician for significant postoperative wound infections requiring prolonged intravenous antibiotics. Approximately 7 months later, the patient underwent a third stage involving resection of the right thigh mass. Her wounds have now resolved and are well healed. This patient represents the second group of body contouring patients with significant comorbitities (Fig. 2).

Peri- and intraoperative precautions

Antibiotic prophylaxis and infection control

For longer, multistage procedures, the risk for infection increases. In part, this can be a consequence of nutritional deficiencies leading to impaired immune states, as well as underlying skin infections, such as candidal colonization manifested by intertrigo, and red rashes between folds. To decrease skin bacterial counts, we advocate washing twice daily with a topical broad-spectrum soap, such as chlorhexidine, starting 3 days before a procedure [16]. Patients are given scrub sponges at their preoperative appointment. Topical and oral antifungals, such as fluconazole, are added to this regimen as appropriate.

Our surgery center strives for a goal of antibiotic prophylaxis administration 1 hour before a procedure [17]. A cephalosporin with good coverage of gram-positive bacteria and skin flora, such as cephazolin, should be dosed and then redosed every 3 and 6 hours during the procedure and adjusted according to the patient's obesity and blood loss. Antibiotic prophylaxis continues for an additional 24 hours postoperatively [18]; however, a common practice among many plastic surgeons is to maintain patients on antibiotics until their drains are removed. Additional measures that we have implemented include intraoperative clipping, rather than shaving, of patients to avoid small cuts and thorough scrubbing with 4% chlorhexidine gluconate during the surgical preparation.

Anesthesia evaluation

Patients who have lost massive amounts of weight may require a complete evaluation by an anesthesiologist because they can be difficult to intubate and sometimes require additional measures, such as fiber-optic intubation or intravenous neck lines. All patients who have lost a massive amount of weight should be questioned regarding a history of gastroesophageal reflux disease, snoring, difficulty sleeping, and whether they have been diagnosed with obstructive sleep apnea to generate an Apnea Screening Index or likelihood of an event [19]. All of these may put the patient at increased risk for aspiration during the procedure. Patients

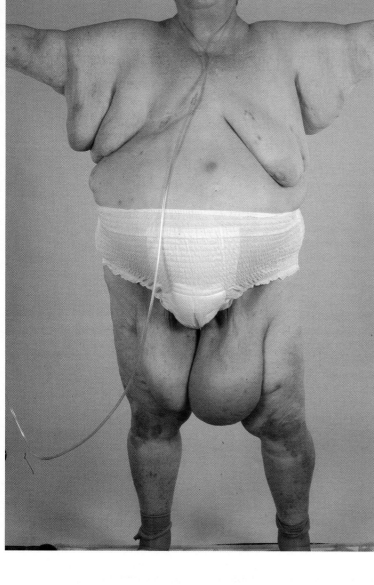

Fig. 2. Preoperative photographs of a 63-year-old woman with a BMI of 54.9 kg/m² who presented with lymphadenomous masses on the inner portion of both thighs. Postoperative complications included COPD exacerbation requiring an ICU stay and significant wound infections requiring prolonged intravenous antibiotics.

who have lost a massive amount of weight have higher rates of sleep apnea than does the general population, and this is characterized by repetitive episodes of upper airway obstruction. Consider using continuous positive airway pressure or an oral appliance while under sedation. Peripheral procedures may be performed safely under an epidural or spinal anesthesia. Monitoring of sleep apnea should continue into the postoperative period, with continuous monitoring of pulse oximetry, ventilation, and cardiac rhythm, and the surgeon should be wary of the respiratory-depressant effects of anesthetics and the overzealous use of narcotics, benzodiazepines, and barbiturates [20]. The decision to supplement with oxygen or

observe with pulse oximetry should have a low threshold.

Positioning

Patients who have lost massive amounts of weight frequently require prone positioning for access to the back and circumferential body contouring; however, this action carries with it risks for neural and vascular compression. Possible described complications include vertebral artery occlusion with associated stroke, vision loss, brachioplexopathies, and shoulder impingement leading to pain and neuropraxias, permanent and temporary [21].

To avoid these sequelae, the head and chest should be in a slightly flexed position with the liberal use of pillows, egg crates, gel mattresses, and foam padding at all nerves and bony prominences, such as the iliac crest, to prevent skin necrosis. The cervical spine should be in a neutral position, and torsion of the spinal cord should be kept to a minimum to prevent trauma to the carotid or vertebral arteries, which are particularly susceptible to subintimal dissection at the atlanto–axial joint. The arterial and venous channels of the eye are at risk for tamponade and collapse, which can lead to temporary or permanent blindness [22,23]. Particular attention to the face is essential; ocular lubricants, taping for eye protection, and a prone pillow or foam cutout that does not compress the nose or ears should be used. Despite meticulous care in set-up, the best reassurance comes from periodic checking of the face throughout the procedure.

The glenohumeral joint of the shoulder should be supported with an axillary roll to prevent subluxation. The arms are susceptible to ulnar, radial, and medial brachial nerve compression and require well-padded boards with foam crates at the elbows and forearms. Once a patient has been placed prone, one always should check the placement of the breasts and nipple position for adequate padding. Pressure is kept off the abdomen in the prone position by placing dual-support rolls from clavicle to pelvic rim. This prevents compression of the chest and the abdominal contents. In the lateral decubitus position, one should place an axillary roll using a rolled blanket or liter bag of saline.

Please note the following illustrative case of multiple complications, including an iatrogenic neurapraxia secondary to malpositioning of the patient intraoperatively for one's initial bariatric procedure. This patient was a bleeding risk secondary to anticoagulation from fen-phen–related valve replacement and had suffered two size-related complications: nerve entrapment and a decubitus ulcer.

Case three

A 58-year-old man had a decrease in BMI from 50.2 kg/m^2 to 35.1 kg/m^2 following gastric bypass. The patient was 5'10" tall, had lost 105 lbs, and presented at 245 lbs. Medical history was significant for insulin-dependent diabetes and aortic valve replacement for which he was anticoagulated on coumadin. After his gastric bypass procedure, the patient sustained a cardiac arrest, underwent a short ICU stay, and subsequently developed a stage 4 gluteal decubitus ulcer. The patient also sustained a left radial nerve and a left common peroneal nerve neuropathy at the fibular head secondary to improper prone positioning without sufficient padding (Fig. 3). Postoperatively, the patient demonstrated an absence of radial nerve function, paralysis of the extensors of the left arm, and paralysis of left foot

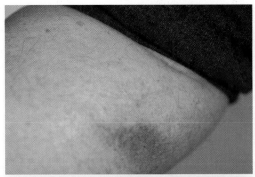
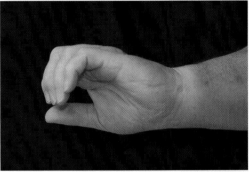

Fig. 3. Postoperative photographs of a 58-year-old man who sustained an iatrogenic nerve paralysis due to improper positioning during a gastric bypass surgery. (*Top*) Postoperative ecchymoses on the patient's dorsal forearm over the radial nerve. (*Bottom*) Note the absence of radial nerve function, with paralysis of the extensors.

dorsiflexion with a burning sensation and paresthesias. Because of the patient's unilateral symptoms, the first assumption was that of stroke, a diagnosis that perpetuated for months until the patient sought a second opinion for the decubitus. After multiple debridements, the patient underwent repair of the decubitus ulcer with a local rotational flap and in a separate procedure, nerve decompression surgery by a peripheral nerve specialist. Immediately postoperatively, the patient developed a hematoma under the pedicle flap secondary to anticoagulation for his fen-phen–related heart valve replacement. This required operative evacuation; however, at 6 months follow-up, the sacral ulcer had healed, and he had regained most muscle function.

Hypothermia

Large amounts of uncovered skin surface during body-contouring procedures can lead to precipitous decreases in core body temperature, contributing to patient instability. Ideally, ambient room temperatures of at least 70°F should be maintained, and as much of the body should be covered as possible. The use of warming air blankets also can be helpful. When turning a patient, warming blankets and sterile towels should be replaced as quickly as possible. Warming equipment for blankets and pre-warmed intravenous fluids should be at or above body temperature before administering to the patient. Our surgical center has found great success with head and foot stockings as well as cutaneous warming devices (Bair Huggers, Augustine Medical, Inc., Eden Prairie, Minnesota) and forced air warming blankets started well before surgery in the preoperative waiting area.

Incisional closure

For all body-contouring procedures, complications have been estimated at around 14.4% for wound problems, 12.9% for seromas, and 2.9% for skin infections [24]. A meticulous multilayered closure is one of the best defenses against incisional dehiscence and infection. Closures should minimize tension. For body lifts, patients should be maintained in a slightly flexed position in bed and during transfers. Postoperatively, patients should not be manipulated until they are completely awake and alert because that is the time at which they can protect themselves. Seromas in potential anatomic planes can be reduced by adequate drain placement and by suture quilting the superficial fascial system to the deep fascial system. When the suspicion of bacterial contamination is high, we have seen some efficacy with using antibacterial triclorsan-coated sutures (Monocryl*Plus and Vicryl*Plus, Ethicon Endo-Surgery, Inc., Cincinnati, Ohio), which inhibited suture colonization [25–27]. After separate suture closures of the fascia, dermis, and finally, epidermis, we advocate using a topical skin adhesive (Dermabond) as a final layer of skin sealant and microbial barrier [28]. This also effectively eliminates the need for dressings that may contribute to dermatitis and skin blistering. Although there is no exact maximal amount of time for body-contouring procedures, a prudent and conservative approach should be taken when deciding how much surgery is safe to perform. There is no single accepted algorithm, but in general, a smaller body mass allows for more procedures to be performed safely at one time. More procedures can be undertaken at one time if a team is used. With a team approach, procedures commonly combined include circumferential body lift with liposuction of thighs, upper body lift with arms, or thigh lift with minor revisions [26]. When combining procedures, performing surgery on multiple distant body parts within a single-stage may predispose patients to problems, because the additional skin exposure increases the likelihood of hypothermia. Surgeries should be kept short enough to prevent significant blood loss and significant hypothermia. A commonly used threshold is to limit surgery to 6 hours,

although this certainly is not universally accepted as a limit. It should be thought of as a guideline, not a standard, which is modifiable by physician and patient comfort levels. Pre- and postoperatively, patients should receive thorough oral education and written instructions about wound care and the signs and symptoms of possible complications.

Postoperative precautions

The use of light-compression garments is an accepted practice for some body-contouring surgeons to prevent seroma and hematoma, despite a paucity of long-term outcome studies. Although we have not found any compromise of skin flaps and support the use of light-compression abdominal binders after liposuction and circumferential torsoplasty, many surgeons believe that the use of compression garments could compromise skin flap blood supply if already made tenuous by extensive undermining and tension closures [27]. If compression garments are used, drain tubes should be moved to avoid pressure necrosis.

Some surgical centers, including ours, are beginning to incorporate ventral hernia repair procedures with body-contouring procedures, such as panniculectomy. This is a safe and effective option in the properly selected patient. We emphasize that the body-contouring surgeon must be aware and vigilant to the theoretic doubling of potential complications with combined surgeries.

Deep vein thrombosis and pulmonary embolism prophylaxis

The risk for deep vein thrombosis (DVT) and pulmonary embolism (PE), estimated at approximately 1.4%, is small, but remains a significant and dreaded complication for the body-contouring surgeon [24]. Certain procedures, such as belt lipectomy, have rates as high as 9.3% [25]. It is important to determine an event probability for a patient based on one's contributing risk factors. Factors associated with thromboembolic phenomena include the use of oral contraceptives, obesity, pregnancy, advanced age, recent surgery, underlying coagulation abnormalities, and prolonged immobilization.

Based on the likelihood of an event, patients may be stratified into four risk categories: low, moderate, high, and highest [29]. In short, the low-risk group consists of patients younger than 40 years of age who are undergoing minor surgery and have no prior risk factors. The moderate-risk group includes patients aged 40 to 60 years with no risk factors who are undergoing minor procedures or patients younger than 40 years who are undergoing a major surgery. High-risk patients are those older than 60 years who are undergoing a minor procedure or those who are older than 40 years, have one risk factor, and are undergoing a major surgery. The highest-risk group are those patients undergoing major surgery after the age of 40 years with a known history of a venous thromboembolic event, hypercoagulable state, hip and knee arthroplasty, major trauma, or spinal cord injury. Recommendations for the prevention of DVTs and PEs is summarized in Fig. 4. Note that certain risks potentiate the effects of other risks. The consequence is that a patient's overall risk may be significantly higher than simply his/her individual risks combined. We have devised a plastic surgery risk-assessment model based on risk profile with appropriate postoperative order selections (Fig. 5) and suggest referencing this system when evaluating a patient initially.

Elastic and mechanical compression stockings or venous foot pumps are suitable for all patients who are undergoing procedures longer than 1 hour and should be applied preoperatively before beginning anesthesia. The best preventative measure is early ambulation; however, if this is not possible, heparin or low molecular weight heparin (LMWH) should be initiated 30 to 60 minutes preoperatively or 12 hours postoperatively for patients in the high- and highest-risk categories [30]. Both agents work through a similar mechanism by inhibiting Xa and IIa (thrombin), important factors in the coagulation cascade. We find that a 12-hour wait before chemo-prophylaxis dosing is the best balance of hematoma risk. LMWH has the added benefits of higher bio-availability, a more predictive dose response, once a day dosing, and a significantly lower incidence of heparin-induced thrombocytopenia [31]. The

surgeon must determine whether this offsets its significant additional expense.

Patients in the highest-risk group may warrant the administration of warfarin; however, this agent has a delayed onset of action compared with LMWH and requires frequent laboratory monitoring. Its role in venous thromboembolic event prophylaxis is limited to patients who refuse LMWH. Current studies are underway to evaluate the effectiveness of new emerging drugs. Fondaparin, a heparin pentasaccharide analog that indirectly inhibits FXa and was approved in 2004 for DVT prophylaxis in orthopedic surgery, has showed early promise in the prevention of thromboembolic events.

The use of aspirin has been shown to decrease the incidence of venous thromboembolism in orthopedic and general surgery patients; however, this reduction was significantly less than that achieved by the previously mentioned agents and did not offset its high-risk profile for gastrointestinal and wound-related bleeding [29].

> The use of epidurals for neuraxial blockade was shown in the orthopedics literature to decrease postoperative mortality and other serious complications, such as DVT, PE, and myocardial infarction [32,33]. Although the overall benefit likely is small, PE after total hip replacement surgery was significantly lower in patients who were given continuous lumbar epidural anesthesia compared with general anesthesia. This research may translate to some indications for its use in the difficult patient who has lost a massive amount of weight.

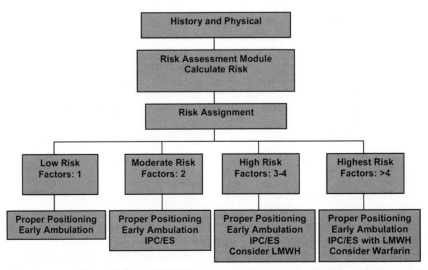

Fig. 4. Algorithm for venous thromboembolism prevention in patients who undergo plastic surgery. ES, elastic compression stockings; IPC, intermittent pneumatic compression stockings; LMWH, low molecular weight heparin. (*From* Davison SP, Venturi ML, Attinger CE, et al. Prevention of venous thromboembolism in the plastic surgery patient. Plast Reconstr Surg 2004;114:43; with permission.)

Step I.   Total = _____

Exposing Risk Factors			
Check the box corresponding to each condition			
1 Factor	**2 Factors**	**3 Factors**	**5 Factors**
Minor surgery ☐	*Major surgery ☐	Previous myocardial infarction ☐	Hip, pelvis, or leg fracture ☐
	Immobilizing plaster cast ☐	Congestive heart failure ☐	Stroke ☐
	Patient confined to bed for > 72 hrs ☐	Severe sepsis ☐	Multiple trauma ☐
	Central venous access ☐	Free flap ☐	Acute spinal cord injury ☐

*Major surgery is defined by the use of general anesthesia or any procedure lasting longer than 1 hour.

Step II.   Total = _____

Predisposing Risk Factors		
Check the box corresponding to each condition		
Clinical Setting	**Inherited**	**Acquired**
Age 40 to 60 (1 Factor) ☐	Any genetic hypercoaguable disorder (3 Factors) ☐	Lupus anticoagulant (3 Factors) ☐
Age > 60 (2 Factors) ☐		Antiphospholipid antibodies (3 Factors) ☐
History of DVT/PE (3 Factors) ☐		Myeloproliferative disorders (3 Factors) ☐
Pregnancy or < 1 month postpartum (1 Factor) ☐		Heparin-induced thrombocytopenia (3 Factors) ☐
Malignancy (2 Factors) ☐		Hyperviscosity (3 Factors) ☐
Obesity > 20% IBW (1 Factor) ☐		Homocystinemia (3 Factors) ☐
Oral contraceptive / hormone replacement therapy (1 Factor) ☐		

Step III.   Total Step I and Step II = _____   Factors

Step IV. Orders

1 Factor	Low risk	Ambulate patient TID ☐
2 Factors	Moderate risk	Intermittent pneumatic compression stockings with elastic compression stockings on at all times when not ambulating ☐
3-4 Factors	High risk	Intermittent pneumatic compression stockings with elastic compression stockings on at all times when not ambulating ☐
> 4 Factors	Highest risk	Intermittent pneumatic compression stockings with elastic compression stockings on at all times when not ambulating ☐ + 1. Enoxaparin (Lovenox) 40mg SQ once daily post op ☐ ***For 1 : Give first dose 12 hours Post Op***

Signature _____   Date/Time _____
Print Name   Pager #

Fig. 5. Plastic surgery venous thromboembolism order form. IBW, ideal body weight; SQ, subcutaneously; TID, three times a day. (*From* Davison SP, Venturi ML, Attinger CE, et al. Prevention of venous thromboembolism in the plastic surgery patient. Plast Reconstr Surg 2004;114:43; with permission.)

Summary

The increase in bariatric procedures will continue to drive the rapidly expanding field of body-contouring surgery. Patients who have undergone bariatric surgery are an inherently difficult patient population whose comorbid conditions must be addressed to perform safe and cautious procedures. The patient who has undergone bariatric surgery and has lost a massive amount of weight is healthier, but still presents risks that should be addressed. As the case studies illustrate, preoperative screening and postoperative care may require consultation and a team approach to manage these deserving patients most safely. DVT prophylaxis is particularly paramount. This systematic review of safety precautions is presented in an effort to reduce the risks and complications of body-contouring surgery.

References

[1] National Institutes of Health Consensus Development Panel. Gastrointestinal surgery for severe obesity. Ann Intern Med 1991;115:956.

[2] Buchwald H, Braunwald E. Bariatric surgery: a systematic review and meta-analysis. JAMA 2004;292:1724.

[3] Mitka M. Surgery useful for morbid obesity, but safety and efficacy questions linger. JAMA 2006; 296:1575–7.

[4] O'Connell JB. Bariplastic surgery. Plast Reconstr Surg 2004;113:1530.

[5] Adler E. After gastric bypass, can body contouring surgery be far behind? Press release: the morning call, KRT News Service, March 21, 2006.

[6] Connolly HM, Crary IL, McGoon MID, et al. Valvular heart disease associated with fenfluramine-phentermine. N Engl J Med 1997;337:581–8.

[7] Aly AS. Approach to the massive weight loss patient. In: Matarasso A, Aly A, Hurwitz D, Lockwood T, editors. Body contouring after massive weight loss. St. Louis (MO): Quality Medical Publishing; 2006. p. 52–6.

[8] Rhode BM, Maclean LD. Vitamin and mineral supplementation after gastric bypass. In: Deitel M, Cowan GSM Jr, editors. Update: surgery for the morbidly obese patient: the field of extreme obesity including laparoscopy and allied care. Toronto: FD Communications; 2000.

[9] Brolin RE, Gorman JH, Gorman RC, et al. Are vitamin B-12 and folate deficiency clinically important after Roux-en-Y gastric bypass? J Gastrointest Surg 1998;2:436.

[10] Dixon JB, Dixon ME, O'Brien PE. Elevated homocysteine levels with weight loss after Lap-Band surgery: higher folate and vitamin B12 levels required to maintain homocysteine level. Int J Obes 2001;25:219.

[11] Hocking MP, Duerson MC, O'Leary JP, et al. Jejunoileal bypass for morbid obesity, late followup in 100 cases. N Engl J Med 1983;308(17): 995–9.

[12] Latham R, Lancaster AD, Covington JF, et al. The association of diabetes and glucose control with surgical-site infections among cardiothoracic surgery patients. Infect Control Hosp Epidemiol 2001;22:607–12.

[13] The Diabetes Control and Complications Trial Research Group. The effect of intensive treatment of diabetes on the development and progression of long-term complications in insulin dependent diabetes mellitus. N Engl J Med 1993;329:977–86.

[14] The Diabetes Control and Complications Trial Research Group. Implications for policy and practice. N Engl J Med 1993;329:1035–6.

[15] Furnary AP, Zerr KJ, Grunkmeier GL, et al. Continuous intravenous insulin infusion reduces the incidence of deep sternal wound infection in diabetic patients after cardiac surgical procedures. Ann Thorac Surg 1999;67:352–62.

[16] Centeno RF, Young VL. Optimal outcome in MWL patients. Shaping Futures 2006;3(2): 1–2.

[17] Mangram AJ, Horan TC, Pearson ML. Guidelines for prevention of surgical site infection. Infect Control Hosp Epidemiol 1999;20:247–8.

[18] Barie PS. Surgical site infections: epidemiology and prevention. Surg Infect (Larchmt) 2002;3: S9–20.

[19] Trott SA, Stool LA, Klein KW. Anesthetic considerations. In: Rohrich RJ, Beran SJ, Kenkel M, editors. Ultrasound-assisted liposuction. St. Louis (MO): Quality Medical Publishing; 1998. p. 74–9.

[20] Practice guidelines for the perioperative management of patients with obstructive sleep apnea. A report by the American Society of Anesthesiologists Task Force on Perioperative Management of Patients with Obstructive Sleep Apnea. Anesthesiology 2006;104(5):1081–93.

[21] Shermak M, Brenda S, Gene DE. Prone positioning precautions in plastic surgery. Plast Reconstr Surg 2006;117(5):15, p 1584–8.

[22] Manfredini M, Ferrante R, Gildone A, et al. Unilateral blindness as a complication of intraoperative positioning for cervical spinal surgery. J Spinal Disord 2000;13:271.

[23] Iverson RE. Patient safety in office-based surgery facilities: I. Procedures in the office-based surgery setting. Plast Reconstr Surg 2002;110: 1337.

[24] Consensus Panel. Examination of the massive weight loss patient and staging considerations. Plast Reconstr Surg 2006;117(1):22S.

[25] Aly AS, Cram AE, Chao M, et al. Belt lipectomy for circumferential truncal excess: the University of Iowa experience. Plast Reconstr Surg 2003; 111(1):398–413.

[26] Shermak MA, Chang D, Magnuson TH, et al. An outcomes analysis of patients undergoing body contouring surgery after massive weight loss. Plast Reconstr Surg 2006;118(4):1026.

[27] Rothenburger S, Spangler D, Bhende S, et al. In vitro antimicrobial evaluation of coated VICRYL* plus antimicrobial suture using zone of inhibition assays. Surg Infect (Larchmt) 2002; 3:s7.

[28] Downey S. The use of fibrin sealant in the prevention of seromas in the massive weight loss patient. [abstract]. Plast Reconstr Surg 2005; 116(Suppl):223.

[29] Geerts WH, Heit JA, Clagett GP, et al. Prevention of venous thromboembolism. Chest 2001; 119(Suppl):132s.

[30] Davison SP, Venturi ML, Attinger CE, et al. Prevention of venous thromboembolism in the plastic surgery patient. Plast Reconstr Surg 2004;114:43e.

[31] Young L, Watson ME. The need for venous thromboembolism (VTE) prophylaxis in plastic surgery. Aesthet Surg J 2006;26(2):157.

[32] Modig J. The role of lumbar epidural anesthesia as antithrombotic prophylaxis in total hip replacement. Acta Chir Scand 1985;151(7):589.

[33] Rodgers A, Walker N, Schug S. Reduction of postoperative mortality and morbidity with epidural or spinal anesthesia: results from overview of randomized trials. BMJ 2000;321:1493.

ELSEVIER
SAUNDERS

CLINICS IN
PLASTIC
SURGERY

Clin Plastic Surg 35 (2008) 185–188

Index

Note: Page numbers of article titles are in **boldface** type.

doi:10.1016/S0094-1298(07)00197-6